BIG FAT LIES

BIG FAT LIES

IS YOUR GOVERNMENT MAKING YOU FAT?

HANNAH SUTTER

Copyright © Go Lower Limited and Hannah Sutter, 2010

The right of Hannah Sutter to be identified as the author of this book has been asserted in accordance with the Copyright, Designs and Patents Act 1988.

First published in 2010 by
Infinite Ideas Limited
36 St Giles
Oxford
OX1 3LD
United Kingdom

www.infideas.com

Reprinted 2010

A CIP catalogue record for this book is available from the British Library

ISBN 978–1–906821–37–1

Brand and product names are trademarks or registered trademarks of their respective owners.

Text designed and typeset by Baseline Arts
Cover designed by Cylinder
Printed in Great Britain by the MPG Books Group, Bodmin and King's Lynn

Acknowledgements

I could not have written this book without the help support and advice of the following individuals:

My husband – who has had to put up with this rant for the past ten years and had to go back to full-time work to allow me the privilege of changing career.

Emily Maguire (nutritionist) – who has helped me in numerous ways but in particular has kindly helped me write the nutrition section.

Dr John Briffa – who has taught me more about the fragility and strength of the human body than anyone.

Professor J. I. Broom – who has carried out research continually, notwithstanding the tide of mainstream thinking.

Professor R. Feinman – for telling me about the horrors of fructose and bringing to life the magic of science.

Drs Michael and Mary Dan Eades – for the most inspiring talk I have ever listened to on the evolution of man's diet.

Garry Taubes – for taking five years out to write the most courageous book on saturated fats ever.

Ken Langdon – for helping me develop my writing skills.

And to everyone who has supported me with my desire to develop natural low-sugar, low-starch products.

Disclaimer

All the ideas here are intended to inform, entertain and provoke your thinking. They're for general information only, and should not be treated as a substitute for medical advice from your own doctor or other healthcare professional. While every effort has been made to provide accurate and up-to-date information, medical science is constantly evolving. Neither the author nor the publisher can be held responsible or liable for any loss or claim arising out of the use, or misuse, of the suggestions made in this book; we don't know your specific circumstances and so we're not suggesting any specific course of action for you to follow. It makes sense for you to weigh up the choices available carefully and to decide what action, if any, you might take; after all, it's your health and it's your life. If in doubt, you should always consult your doctor for individualised health and medical advice.

Although the contents of this book were checked at the time of going to press, the world keeps moving as does the world wide web. This means we can't guarantee the contents of any of the websites mentioned in the text.

Contents

Introduction

How would you feel if you found out that it was the government that had made you fat? Would you want to change the government, sue for damages or simply accept an apology? Well, get ready to make that decision.

For the past thirty years the government has told us to eat less and do more and we, as a nation, have done just that. We eat 500 fewer calories a day than we did in the slim 1970s; we do more exercise now than we did under Thatcher, but we are still getting fatter and fatter. To make matters worse, the messages of eating less and doing more are accelerating the growth of obesity in the UK.

The 'eat less, do more' message has been blasted out by almost everyone, following the government line on the assumption that this must be right. The real underlying meaning of this message, for those who have not picked up on it, is that anyone who is fat is that way because they are greedy and lazy!

However, did you know that this message has never been proven using randomised clinical trials? In other words, there has never been any form of proper testing done, and if this message of 'eat less, do more' was taken to a court it simply would not stand up to cross-examination. We expect all other forms of medical advice to be properly tested, so why do we accept this second-rate attitude to diet when the biggest health crisis in Britain today is without doubt linked to it? In fact, we only started to get really fat since governments started promoting the current health messages. During the past ten years we have actually increased the amount of exercise we are doing and more of us are calorie counting than ever before. Sadly, the government, through the Food Standards Agency (FSA), is repeating the same health advice with complete disregard to the fact that it is not working – even though we do know that people are complying with the message more and more.

This book has been written to set the record straight and point the finger at the real culprit in the biggest crime of this decade. The criminals on trial are not the obese or the diabetics who have been blamed for being fat, but the government which has made our nation obese with 'expert knowledge' that is, sadly, not based on robust science. Obesity and diabetes, for a significant percentage of the population, are inevitable consequences of the advice given out by the Food Standards Agency. The co-defendant in the dock with the government is starch. While we have all be blaming fat as the 'murderer', starch has been quietly knocking us off while we are being told that it is good for us.

Ultimately, finding out who is guilty and demanding accountability has always been the expertise of lawyers, and now it is again time for a lawyer to expose the biggest lies of our generation. More people die each day as a result of the big starch lie than are killed in Iraq or Afghanistan.

So, find out why we are fat today and discover how to solve your weight problem the most natural and honest way without the need for bariatric surgery, shakes, drugs, hunger or exercise...

Ask two simple questions

What do lawyers do? They ask questions and keep asking questions until they get a satisfactory answer. Lawyers are trained to look at facts objectively and dissect information to find out the truth. They are skilled at seeing inconsistencies and proficient at sniffing out bullshit. A lot of other professionals hate lawyers because, without apparent expert knowledge, they can show a misdemeanour simply through the use of cross-examination. When a doctor is charged with medical negligence it is the lawyer who will prove whether the medical negligence occurred. The lawyer will cross-examine the expert doctors looking for the error or the inconsistency. And nothing makes lawyers happier than when they find a liar.

It seems a long time ago that I was a partner in an international law firm practising corporate law. My up-to-eighteen-hour days were spent in offices reading and negotiating long contracts on behalf of businessmen, looking for lies and inconsistencies. Finding one inconsistency could save a client literally millions. If asked, I would have assured anyone that this was my career for life. It was extremely well paid and really interesting at times, especially when the deals were difficult or complicated. However everything changed for me in 2002 because of a minor incident: two fat men got thin.

At the time I was acting on behalf of a company that was preparing to float on the London Stock Market. The transaction took a couple of months to complete and during the six-to-eight-week run-up to the float two fat bankers shed, between them, about six stones. Every few days they would turn up at my office a little slimmer. Every visit their trousers were a little baggier. In fact, the flotation team became far more interested in their physical progress than in the client and its fundraising.

At the end of the process I took these two elegant and slim men out for lunch and asked them for the secret. Was it the no-food diet (often called the cabbage-soup diet) or the marathon diet (that is the one when you have to run a marathon each day), or was it something more obvious like the 'eat less and do more' diet?

They were delighted to share the secret of their success. They explained that they had taken the advice of a private consultant in Harley Street who had put them on a ketogenic diet. No exercise was required and they could eat unlimited quantities of food – the perfect diet for bankers who loved lunches and dinners but hated the gym.

Over lunch they shared the fifty-guinea secret. Eat as much meat, fish, eggs, nuts and seeds as you want and then have your daily portions of green vegetables and berries. Occasionally snack on cheese and have a glass of red wine every day. Because of the involvement of a doctor they were having cholesterol and other health checks on a regular basis and the results were impressive.

After lunch I wandered back to the office to pack my bags and return to Edinburgh where I spent the weekends with my family. For the whole of the journey from Bank Station to my house in Edinburgh all I could think about was what these bankers had told me. Like almost every woman over the age of thirty-five, I worried about weight and fat. I had speed-read all the books from the *Raw Food Diet* through to the *Rosemary Conley Hip and Thigh Diet* but none had told me to do anything like these bankers had done.

All the books I had read by dieticians and other diet experts had one very simple message: eat less, and eat less fat. Fill yourself with grains and fibre and small amounts of lean protein with lots of vegetables and fruit. But I had seen, before my eyes, two fat men get thin doing something quite different.

The lawyer in me saw, quite obviously, that there was something not completely consistent. The only thing I knew is that fat is simply stored energy. Surely the questions that I needed to answer were how do we become fat – what is the bodily process that makes us turn the food we eat into saturated fat on our bodies – and how can we use up body fat?

These may seem like simple questions to answer. The standard diet books simply said we get fat because we eat too much, and to use up the fat we need to do more and eat less – but whichever way I looked at the fat bankers, there was clearly an inconsistency. In fact, the more I thought about the inconsistency the more times I was reminded about all those friends or colleagues who had religiously followed low-fat , low calorie diets and failed either in the short term or put the weight back on later. The weird and counter-intuitive diet of eating lots and doing nothing did seem to work extremely well.

Once I was back in Edinburgh I started to cross-examine my GP husband, Andy. Frankly, his response was hopeless. He admitted that he couldn't remember the science on weight gain but told me that it was definitely to do with too many calories. In other words, if you eat more calories than you burn your body will have to turn the excess calories into stored energy, which is saturated fat. So in his 'expert' opinion being fat was simply about eating too much. I then explained the paradox of these fat men who had become slim while eating a lot of food and doing no exercise.

His response was that they must be lying and went back to reading his surfing magazine. After several attempts at further questioning, Andy gave me the number of a cardiologist in Edinburgh he thought might know more. It turned out to be a kind act.

Meeting David Northridge at a friend's house some weeks later was a memorable moment. He was the first person to explain some basic biochemistry to me. As a consultant cardiologist in Edinburgh, David had lots of experience in dealing with people who were struggling to lose weight and who had unpleasant arteries clogged with bad cholesterol and were fat.

Over dinner he confirmed that the banker's diet did make sense because of the combination of foods that they were eating. What David went on to explain to me, in very basic language, was that the doctrine that we get fat because we eat too much – and in particular because we eat too much fat – was not based on robust science. While common sense would seem to support this theory, actual science had not been particularly supportive. He made the comparison with medieval men believing that the world was flat. He said the belief that fat and calories make you fat looks and sounds perfectly reasonable but is an illusion, as the fat bankers had shown. The critical trigger in the human metabolism for turning food into fat is the hormone insulin and without insulin it is impossible to gain fat no matter what or how much you eat. So, in a nutshell, gaining weight has less to do with how much you eat but more to do with what you eat and how your body deals with your insulin response.

David's answer to my fat questions was that to gain fat you need to produce insulin, and the more insulin you produce the more likely it is that you will gain fat. David then explained that the only really effective way to use up body fat (i.e. lose fat) is to make the body go into a natural state of ketosis which forces it to burn off the body fat it has stored. In his opinion, the banker's diet made perfect sense because it did two things at once. First, the diet was unlikely to require a significant release of insulin and, second, it was likely to force the body to go into ketosis and burn its body fat. He also assured me that this process was quite natural and safe. He even said, 'We are designed to do just this.'

This was fascinating. After an hour with David and a further hour on Amazon buying books I had got myself sucked into the subject of nutrition and, in particular, insulin. Within weeks I had read everything from *Dr Atkins' New Diet Revolution* to *Protein Power* and *The South Beach Diet*. The books all referred to published science to back up their statements and all of them saw insulin as the key to solving the obesity crisis. Each of these books made a mockery of calorie counting and low-fat diets, as had the two fat bankers.

Against this backdrop, I became more and more aware of the messaging in the public domain on calories and fat. Again and again the only message I could hear from the mouths of our 'experts' was 'eat less, eat less fat and exercise more'. To be honest, the lawyer in me was horrified. Just like everyone, I knew someone who had a significant weight problem and who was desperately eating lots of starch (high-fibre versions), much less fat and sweating at the gym with no success. Why did they not know about insulin and the impact of insulin on their metabolism? Why had no one told them about the poor evidence against fatty foods, currently the main criminal in the offence of obesity?

A lawyer is trained to sniff out inconsistencies and where possible seek out the truth and all I could see around me was porky-pies being punted to the public as facts. I couldn't actually believe it was possible to make such grandiose statements about what to eat based on such dubious evidence. With so many people significantly overweight it was like watching massive abuse taking place. Our government was actually making people fat and making fat people fatter with the advice they were handing out. At the same time the experts were repeating the mantra set out by the government and, just to jolly things along, the food industry was producing more and more products complying with government guidelines which were being bought by more and more people...

After six months of reading various books written by various doctors I was completely obsessed with the insulin message, and it was all I could think and talk about. I even got friends to follow low-insulin-impact diets and watched the inches fall away. Even at work, all I ever talked about in the canteen with my colleagues was food and this new way of eating.

At this time the Atkins diet was at its peak, but one of the main challenges was the lack of snacks for people looking to keep their insulin levels low while eating natural foods. I spent many a lunchtime walking up and down Cheapside in the City of London going in and out of food stores, from Holland and Barrett to M&S, looking for really healthy snacks that wouldn't cause an insulin response. The choice was either highly processed and unnatural snacks made by diet companies or natural snacks that would cause insulin levels to rise.

I saw the opportunity and grabbed it. After much debate with clients and colleagues, I decided to make a change. I had spent seventeen great years in law working with some of the UK's best entrepreneurs but now I wanted to do it for myself. So I resigned and set up golower to make natural, high-protein, low-starch/low-sugar food. On 4 July I handed in my notice and flew home to tell Andy the good news. He wasn't too impressed, as it meant that he had to go back to full-time work while I would go to work in the kitchen. From riches to poverty in just one resignation letter!

THE REAL DIET EXPERT

The two simple questions which took me from law to food were:
◆ How do we become fat – what is the bodily process that makes us turn the food we eat into saturated fat on our bodies?
◆ How can we use up body fat?

Most people believe that the answers to these simple and rather obvious questions are that:
◆ We are fat because we have consumed too many calories compared with the amount of calories that we have expended, and therefore the excess calories have turned to fat
◆ To lose the fat we need to eat less and burn the excess fat to replace the missing calories from our diet.

So the obvious solution is that we must eat fewer calories and do more exercise. By eating less and doing more at the same time we can create a sufficient deficit between our energy in and our actual expenditure. This is the view expressed on the following expert websites.

Diabetes UK:
> You need to look at how much you're eating a day, and look at how much you're putting on your plate and see where you need to reduce the calories... It might be helpful to ask your diabetes nurse if you can have an appointment with the dietician and get individual advice on healthy eating.

The Food Standards Agency:
> When someone is obese, it means they have put on weight to the point that it could seriously endanger their health. This is caused by a combination of eating too many calories and not doing enough physical activity.

NHS Direct:
> Physical activity increases the amount of calories you use up. The more exercise you do, the more calories you will burn. This means that if you increase the amount of exercise you do without increasing your food intake, the extra energy needed will be taken from your stored body fat and you will lose weight.

BBC Health:
> How to lose weight.
> Losing weight depends on energy balance. If you consume more energy from food and drink than you burn through maintaining your body's functions (metabolism) and physical activity, you'll gain weight. Cutting calories by reducing how much you eat and drink, and increasing how much physical activity you do, will make you lose weight. If you reduce your daily energy intake to around 500 calories (kcal) below your energy requirements, you'll lose about 0.5kg (1lb) a week. This is a sensible rate of weight loss.

British Dietetic Association:
> Did you know? One pound of fat contains 3,500 calories, so to lose 1lb a week you need a deficit of 500 calories a day.

OK, all well and good, but I had seen two fat men eat loads of calories and, without exercising, lose weight and inches fast. David, the cardiologist, had explained to me why the bankers' diet worked but I needed to beef up on my knowledge so, once I had negotiated my 'garden leave', I attended the first ever conference on low-carb, high-protein diets in Denver, USA.

By the time I arrived in Denver the conference had started. Ignoring the jet lag, I went straight into meetings. One of the first seminars I attended was called 'The paradox of more calories and faster weight loss'. Professor Feinman, head of biochemistry at Sunny Downstate University, NY, gave the lecture.

His paper was in response to a violent outcry in the US following the publication of several peer-reviewed studies[1] comparing different diets. The weird outcome that shocked a great many experts was that, for some reason, the group that lost the most weight and inches in their comparative research were eating more calories than other groups in some cases. There was no exercise element to affect the outcome.

The studies had not been intended to produce these results but they did. They compared low-fat diets to low-carb diets and, notwithstanding 500 more calories a day in some of the low-carb groups, the low-carbers beat the low-fat groups in terms of weight and inch loss.

Two hours later I understood why this outcome should have been anticipated. Professor Feinman explained why the measuring of food by reference to calories is fundamentally flawed, for many reasons. One of these fundamental flaws are the rules of, would you believe, thermodynamics. By the end of the seminar it was quite clear that anyone with A-level physics could have explained why fewer calories would not necessarily mean greater weight loss. So the simple rules of thermodynamics and the various studies tell us that calorie counting is not based on science, even if it sounds intuitive and logical. The amount of food you eat will naturally have an impact on your metabolism and size, but the actual calorific quantity is a very small part of a very complex equation, which we will explore in Chapter Four.

After Professor Feinman, I listened to several other doctors speak. By the end of my first day in Denver I realised that putting the sole reason for weight loss and weight gain on the role of calories in the diet reflects a very poor understanding of human biochemistry as well as the rules of thermodynamics.

I went to bed that night with three clear messages:
- Eating fewer calories is founded on a fundamental misunderstanding that the body burns calories of different types equally
- The conversion from food to fat in the human body is not simple
- The conversion of fat back into usable energy is not that obvious either.

THE NEXT STEP

The Denver trip was the real launch of my nutrition journey and it will stay with me forever. I am delighted to say that many of the doctors and specialists I met way back at the 2004 conference are still friends and associates today. Armed with more science and a long reading list I returned to the UK to really start golower.

Into the kitchen I went, to develop a range of products that complied with nutritional requirements to help people lose weight fast – the natural way. Unlike the competition, I wanted to develop foods that worked with our natural biochemistry rather than ones which were simply low in calories. I wanted my foods to do everything that I learned from the specialists I had met and listened to in Denver.

One of the most memorable talks at the conference was by Drs Michael and Mary Dan Eades who asked the diet-food industry to only make foods that are free of artificial ingredients and are also fundamentally healthy – that is, rich in vitamins and minerals and all the other nutrients needed for a healthy life. In other words, weight-loss products should still comply with the very highest standards; if anything, diet food should be more nutritious as that is key to helping people solve their weight problem.

I took this message to heart and set about producing products that complied with all these standards. This meant that I couldn't use any sugars including fructose, but also that I needed to avoid artificial sweeteners like aspartame, polyols, saccharine and so forth. It meant not using artificial additives to make things last longer and not using artificial flavours or colours: in fact, going back to basics.

The journey had started, and I began to make great diet food based on robust scientific evidence and with the principle of no compromise.

Summing up

The best experts for uncovering bullshit are lawyers, even when they are not qualified in the relevant discipline – for example, medical negligence.

Two fat men got thin and stayed thin by eating lots of food and doing no exercise.

There is a contrary opinion on how to lose fat which is not based on calorie counting. It is supported by peer-reviewed science but this opinion is not being shared with those who are struggling to lose weight.

The biological processes of becoming fat and then turning body fat back into usable energy are not straightforward.

In peer-reviewed scientific trials, eating fewer calories was not linked to improved inch or weight loss.

Fat facts

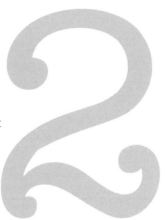

Whenever you start an investigation into an inconsistency you start with the facts that you can find. So before I explain why the government has made us fat we need to look closely at the government facts or statistics. Like all loud-mouthed people, the government gives the game away without even meaning to.

So before you put the book down, saying 'We all know that we're getting fatter blah, blah, blah', do read this chapter because you'll find out some really interesting facts and statistics that have been hidden away in various reputable and well-publicised government and quasi-governmental reports. I can only presume that either no one bothered to read the statistics or someone, somewhere doesn't fancy a debate about them.

OBESITY STATISTICS

Let's start from the top.

By 2010, 13 million people in the UK will be obese – that's from the Department of Health Report 'Forecasting Obesity to 2010' of July 2006. In the same year, 2006, and nearly every year since then, the NHS also produced a report called 'Statistics on Obesity, Physical Activity and Diet: England' (NHS Reports). (You'll find a short definition of obese and overweight by reference to the BMI – body mass index calculation – in the notes to this chapter.[1])

So over the past five years there has been a great deal of research into our population and the obesity epidemic. The main findings from the various NHS studies can be summarised as follows:

◆ In the years between 1993 and 2005 the proportion of men classed as obese increased from 13.2% to 23.1%. That's a rate of growth of 75% in just twelve years

◆ In the same period the proportion of women classed as obese increased from 16% to 24.8%. That is a growth of 55 % in twelve years
◆ Our calorific intake between the years 1974 and 2004 decreased by 20%
◆ We are also eating more fruit and vegetables – an estimated 20% increase
◆ We are doing more exercise than we were in 1997, approximately 25% more
◆ During the period between 1993 and 2005 there was no significant increase in the number of people who were overweight.

Now, before you yawn and close this book you may want to reread the above with the following conclusions in mind:
◆ We are eating less
◆ We are eating more foods that are associated with a healthy diet
◆ There has been an average increase in obesity of 65% over the past twelve to thirteen years. The actual number of people who are overweight has not increased, but those who are overweight are becoming obese faster and faster.

So what is actually happening is that, for a significant portion of the population, we are seeing a rapid increase in the speed at which they move from being overweight to obese. The difference between being overweight and obese is significant, as obesity brings with it significant health-related issues from diabetes to heart disease and cancer. As you consider this you need to remember that we are all eating fewer calories now than we did before.

This is all very interesting, but let's now add a little fuel to the fire.

FAT TUMMIES AND THE MISLEADING PURSUIT OF THE BMI (BODY MASS INDEX)

What is not immediately apparent from the government statistics is that we are getting fatter around the middle.

The proportion of adults who have fat tummies has grown from 23% to 37% in just twelve to thirteen years,[2] which is an overall increase of a whopping 60%. This may seem irrelevant but this is one of the biggest single pieces of critical information. In the appendix you can look at the raw data straight from the horse's mouth.

Does it matter if we are getting fatter round the waist? Yes, it does, and when I found this out it made me weep. So while our government witters on about BMI it has been shown that waist circumference (or abdominal obesity or fat tummy) is the biggest indicator of heart health and doubles the odds of having a heart attack.[3] It is also a key indicator of diabetes and other health issues.[4]

Let me just summarise. Being fat around the tummy is completely different from having a fat bum. Your BMI tells you whether you are big by making a comparison of weight and height, but it does not really tell you if you are fat and nor does it tell you if you are fat in an unhealthy way. The BMI is ultimately a poor indicator of health and can be misleading. For example, the BMI of most of professional rugby players would mean they were classed as overweight or obese, but clearly they are not fat. They are muscular – which is positive.

While there has been a virtually continuous onslaught by scientists desperately trying to show that the most important indicator to health is waist measurement, all our government wants to talk about is the BMI which has been acknowledged as misleading. Measuring waist size accurately may be a little tricky, but at least the information gained is useful.

Keep in mind the following:
◆ Some of us have tummies that are growing at an exponential rate
◆ Fat tummies are the real indicator of health
◆ The massive increase in fat tummy growth took off in the 1990s when the government first started really hammering on about a low-calorie, healthy, balanced diet.

EXERCISE STATISTICS

So some of us (about 40% of the UK's adult population) are eating less but developing fatter tummies. It may be a reasonable assumption that the problem is down to a lack of exercise – if you believe that it is all about calories in and calories out. This is exactly what the government has presumed, but where is the evidence?

In the same NHS report which shows that our calorific intake is going down there are also tables showing that our exercise levels have stayed approximately the same for the past seven years and, if anything, have risen slightly. You'll find some details in the appendix.

There are no statistics for what came before 1997, but there are studies in Europe that have consistently shown that exercise does not appear to have any significant impact on our size. While this may surprise many of us, it has been known by many experts in the world of obesity for some time, and they include Sir Neville Rigby who was chairman of the European Obesity Task Force for many years. Closer to home, there is a large-scale study being carried out by a professor at Plymouth University looking at the impact of exercise on childhood obesity and he, surprisingly, has so far found that exercise has little, if any, impact.[5]

Summing up

Working from the government statistics and the 2008 NHS report we know that we are:

◆ Eating less
◆ Eating more vegetables and fruit – closer to the balanced diet
◆ Doing more exercise.

The same report tells us that a significant percentage of the population is getting fatter more quickly. While the number of overweight people is not significantly increasing, the number of overweight people becoming obese is rising more quickly.

Therefore we've been taking the advice we have been given, but it is not working for some of us. It could be argued that the advice given may well be accelerating the problem for those people who are becoming obese.

What is most notable about the statistics is the rise in fat tummies. A fat tummy is recognised as a key health indicator and associated with insulin resistance and other health problems.

When a patient is sick and the medicine prescribed is not working, the worst thing to do is to keep giving the same medicine. Having said that, doctors did use leeches for many hundreds of years as a remedy for many ills before it was pointed out to them that they were not working very well...

What the government experts say

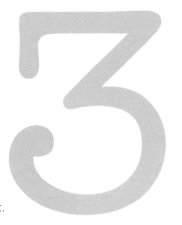

Having looked at the facts, a prosecution lawyer then starts looking closely at the statements made by the defence. In this case the defendant is the UK government and it has set out its statement on the website of the Food Standards Agency (FSA) which is a non-ministerial department of the government. The FSA deals with all the following matters:

◆ Nutrition
◆ Food safety and hygiene
◆ Labelling and packaging
◆ GM and novel food
◆ Food industries
◆ Enforcement
◆ Research and science.

In the Nutrition section, the Agency gives guidelines on what to eat. This is the Eatwell website:[1] 'For advice on healthy eating, visit our eatwell site. It's packed with information and tips on eating a healthy balanced diet.'

This section starts with this simple statement:

A healthy balanced diet contains a variety of foods including plenty of fruit and vegetables, plenty of starchy foods such as wholegrain bread, pasta and rice, some protein-rich foods such as meat, fish, eggs and lentils, and some dairy foods. It should also be low in fat (especially saturated fat), salt and sugar.

And you are then directed to the eatwell plate – 'The eatwell plate makes healthy eating easier to understand by showing the types and proportions of foods we need to have a healthy and well balanced diet.'

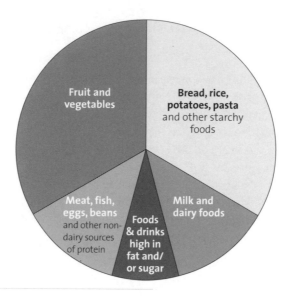

Figure 3.1 – A representation of the eatwell plate

The website goes on to say:

> The eatwell plate shows how much of what you eat should come from each food group. This includes everything you eat during the day, including snacks. So, try to eat:
>
> ◆ plenty of fruit and vegetables
> ◆ plenty of bread, rice, potatoes, pasta and other starchy foods – choose wholegrain varieties whenever you can
> ◆ some milk and dairy foods
> ◆ some meat, fish, eggs, beans and other non-dairy sources of protein
> ◆ just a small amount of foods and drinks high in fat and/or sugar.
>
> Look at the eatwell plate to see how much of your food should come from each food group. You don't need to get the balance right at every meal. But try to get it right over time such as a whole day or week.

In other words, the simple message is base your meals on starch and vegetables and fruit. The remaining third of your meals should be primarily divided between protein and dairy, with a small place for sugar and fatty foods.

The British Dietetic Association (BDA) also suggest that people should look to the FSA for guidelines on eating well: 'All you need to do is eat sensibly, choosing a range of foods in the correct proportions. The Food Standards Agency (FSA) eatwell plate is made up of five food groups – simply choose a variety of foods from each group.'

I must admit that it is a novel idea that there are five good groups as I was under the impression that we had three – protein, fat and carbohydrates. Now let's dig a bit deeper. Here are the FSA's top tips on eating well:

- Base your meals on starchy foods
- Eat lots of fruit and vegetables
- Eat more fish
- Cut down on sugar and fat
- Try to eat less salt
- Get active [Since when was this an eating tip?]
- Drink plenty of water
- Don't skip breakfast.

You may note that protein is not important to our diet, according to the FSA. Again this is something to remember when we come to the definition of what the human diet really needs to be.

The NHS website is also a provider of expert knowledge on how to eat, and the eatwell plate is replicated almost identically on it:

A well-balanced diet includes food from the five main food groups. These are:

- bread, cereal (including breakfast cereals) and potatoes (starchy foods)
- fruit (including fresh fruit juice) and vegetables
- meat and fish
- milk and dairy foods, and
- fat and sugar.

No difference there.

Both websites also provide advice on how to lose weight. The NHS says:
> The recommended daily calorie intake varies depending on how old you are. For the average adult this is about 2,000 per day (women) and 2,500 per day (men). These calories should be made up of foods from the main food groups. *If you're trying to lose weight, you could start by eating 500 less calories per day.* [My emphasis.]

And the FSA sums it up as follows:
> Whenever we eat more than our body needs, we put on weight. This is because the energy we don't use up is stored in our body, usually as fat. *Even small amounts of surplus energy each day can lead to weight gain* [again, my emphasis]. So if you want to lose some weight, you might want to look at ways of:
> ◆ making sure you only eat as much food as you need
> ◆ improving the balance of your diet
> ◆ getting more active.

If you then turn your attention to the British Nutrition Foundation (BNF), they believe that the energy density of food is the solution: 'Energy (or calories) per gram of food may provide a key to tackling the alarming rise in obesity.' This is really a variation of the same basic message.

The BDA also have advice on how to shed those pounds in the face of the obesity crisis, and they too reflect the views of the FSA. Their suggestion is really simple. Reduce your calorie intake by 500 calories a day and do some exercise.

In summary, therefore, the FSA leads the way on all matters relating to healthy eating. It states that the eatwell plate is the best dietary guideline for everyone in the UK, and that to lose weight you should:
> ◆ Eat less
> ◆ Eat a balanced diet according to the eatwell plate.

(For some reason they add the exercise message here but, of course, this is not an eating tip.)

Having set out the 'right' way to eat, the FSA has also then brought in the traffic-light labelling guidelines to help the consumer buy food according to the eatwell plate. The traffic-light system has been designed so that the consumer can eat without thinking and feel safe in the guidance given by these experts.

Summing up

The FSA website is used as the reference point for all other health websites including those of the NHS and the BDA. The FSA is telling us to:

◆ Eat a healthy diet according to the eatwell plate
◆ Eat less
◆ Exercise more.

As we've seen, we know that people are doing more and eating less, and eating more fruit and vegetables.

Notwithstanding increasing compliance with these messages, the obesity numbers are growing and the speed of growth is accelerating.

There have been no randomised trials carried out to test whether the advice given by the FSA will bring about the results it wants.

Big fat lies

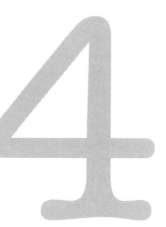

The cross-examination of any defendant is the longest and most difficult part of any court action and sometimes members of the jury lose sight of where the lawyer is taking the argument. We can all remember court-room dramas which turn upon one or two key questions at the right moment to illustrate the deceit.

So, just like Perry Mason, we need to start with the defendant's own statement and then show why it is based on a fallacy.

The key statements of the FSA are:
◆ Eat less
◆ Eat a healthy diet (according to the eatwell plate)
◆ Exercise more.

Each one of these statements is misleading and, for those people who are obese or overweight, it can be shown that these statements are accelerating their obesity problem. So we have three big fat lies:
◆ Big fat lie 1 – eat less and eat fewer calories
◆ Big fat lie 2 – eat a diet according to the eatwell plate
◆ Big fat lie 3 – do more.

BIG FAT LIE 1 – EAT LESS

Eating less can mean many things but for the FSA (the government), it is about two things, eating less food and eating fewer calories.

'Eat less' does seem obvious, and yet we know from many studies that the actual amount of calories consumed did not decide the diet outcome; remember the group eating more calories lost more fat.[1] We know from the NHS Reports of 2006 and 2008 and a separate independent study in 2005 that we eat less today than we did when we were slimmer in the 1970s.[2]

Notwithstanding this empirical science and government-collected statistics, the intuitive certainty of the message of calorie counting continues to dominate the thinking of our government. As a perfect example of this continuing faith in calorie counting, last year our government launched a campaign to encourage restaurants to start providing calorie details for each meal – just like the processed-food companies do. Dawn Primarolo, then the Public Health Minister, said that she 'wanted to see more companies and more outlets help even more people live healthier lives ... by providing the calorie count in their takeaway and eating-out meals'.

The paradox doesn't stop with the statistics or the empirical evidence. While our waistbands have been growing over the past ten years, our awareness of calorie counting has also grown. The latest data from the British Market Research Bureau, at the time of writing, shows that since 1998 the number of adults who think about food in terms of calories has doubled. When you read this, in the context of the rising obesity numbers in the same period, you do wonder what further calorie counting is going to do for our well-being.

You might jump to the seemingly obvious conclusion that the problem is exercise or the lack of exercise, but hold your horses and put that thought to one side for a moment – or at least until later in this cross-examination.

While calorie counting does tell us the amount of energy there is in food, it does not give us a whole heap of other critical information which will affect our weight far more than simple energy intake. Calorie counting does not tell us about the impact of food on the following:
- Insulin response
- Satiety – feeling full
- Sustainability – practicality
- Metabolic rate
- Nutrient famine
- Thermodynamics – calorie burn.

Each one of these issues makes a mockery of calorie counting. To help you follow the debate I have set out below a list of different foods equal to 100 calories. Keep this in mind as you work through this chapter because it will highlight the complete stupidity of measuring food simply by its calorific intake and then building a whole nation's eating habits on this limited and frequently misleading information.

◆ 1 boiled egg
◆ 40g bran flakes
◆ 1.5 Brazil nuts
◆ 1 chocolate biscuit
◆ 100g kidney beans
◆ 120g new potatoes
◆ 500g spinach
◆ 60g steak
◆ 36 strawberries.

INSULIN RESPONSE
Calorie counting does not tell you what the insulin response to food is, and yet the role of insulin in human metabolism is fundamental to understanding whether or not we will gain weight regardless of calorific input. To understand this we need a short lesson in biochemistry. Don't give up now because if there is one message to take from this book then this is it.

A SHORT LESSON IN BIOCHEMISTRY
In the most simplistic terms, when we eat food our bodies break down the starch in the food into glucose molecules in the body and absorb them into the bloodstream. As the food is converted into glucose there is a natural rise in blood-glucose levels and this will trigger the release of a hormone called insulin. Insulin then exerts its metabolic effect by binding itself to specific receptors on cell membranes that allow glucose to be brought into muscle and several other target tissues. Once the glucose gets into muscle it is utilised to provide energy via a process called glycolysis. If the glucose is not expended as energy – because you are sitting at the computer, for example – then insulin will transport the

excess glucose for storage. We need to store excess glucose because too much glucose in our blood can cause blindness, circulation problems, coma and other nasties over time.

There are two ways to store glucose. A small amount of glucose can be stored as glycogen in the liver; the excess will synthesise triglycerides and eventually be stored as fat. Figure 4.1 shows the process diagramatically.

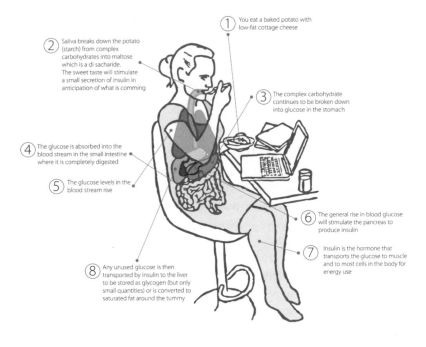

1 You eat a baked potato with low-fat cottage cheese

2 Saliva breaks down the potato (starch) from complex carbohydrates into maltose which is a di sacharide. The sweet taste will stimulate a small secretion of insulin in anticipation of what is comming

3 The complex carbohydrate continues to be broken down into glucose in the stomach

4 The glucose is absorbed into the blood stream in the small intestine where it is completely digested

5 The glucose levels in the blood stream rise

6 The general rise in blood glucose will stimulate the pancreas to produce insulin

7 Insulin is the hormone that transports the glucose to muscle and to most cells in the body for energy use

8 Any unused glucose is then transported by insulin to the liver to be stored as glycogen (but only small quantities) or is converted to saturated fat around the tummy

Figure 4.1 – The role of insulin in the digestion of starch

So the conversion process of food to human fat is ultimately triggered by the release of insulin, forcing the body to start collecting excess glucose as fat. This is really important, because without insulin you simply can't get fat. If this still doesn't make much sense, let me give you a real example given to me by a diabetic expert. It helped me understand what was going on.

A type 1 diabetic is a person who has no insulin due to the complete failure of the pancreas. If someone with type 1 diabetes does not take insulin lots of terrible things will happen but, for the purpose of this chapter, the key thing that you would see is that they would fail to gain fat even if they were eating suet for breakfast, lard for lunch and sugar for dinner. Without insulin you cannot convert glucose to fat; it won't happen. What actually does happen is that your body simply can't make the conversion from glucose to fat.

So, what we now know is that insulin is very important for helping us to use glucose for energy (the first part of the process in Figure 4.1 – transportation of glucose to muscles, etc.) but it will, if you have too much glucose or if you overproduce insulin, create fat. The overproduction of insulin accelerates fat gain even if you are eating less. If someone constantly overproduces insulin they can lose their sensitivity to it, and this is known as being 'insulin resistant'. If you develop insulin resistance you will produce even more insulin.

One of the key indicators of over production of insulin or insulin resistance is a fat tummy,[3] and you may recall that one of the key features of our obesity epidemic is the significant increase in fat tummies. This obvious link is really important to keep in mind. We'll come on to over-production of insulin and insulin resistance in further detail later.

Different foods trigger different amounts of insulin regardless of the calorie count.[4] A person could eat 200 calories of steak and have a low insulin response or 100 calories of starch and have a greater insulin response. Remember that the release of insulin and the amount of insulin released defines, to some extent, how much fat you are likely to collect in your body.

Let's look at the anticipated insulin response, in a healthy person, of the following foods:

Food	Calories (approx)	Insulin Index
1 boiled egg	100	low
40g bran flakes	100	medium
1.5 Brazil nuts	100	low
1 chocolate biscuit	100	high
100g kidney beans	100	medium
120g new potatoes	100	high
500g spinach	100	low
60g steak	100	low
36 strawberries	100	low

Table 4.1 – Insulin response

So there's no correlation between the amount of calories something contains and the anticipated insulin response. While calories (a measurement of energy) should appear to be equal to the amount or impact of blood sugar, in reality that is not how the body operates. For example, fat is high in calorific value – which is one of the reasons we are told to reduce our fat intake – but fats tend to have a low insulin response unless they are man-made trans fats or mixed with starch or sugar. Therefore, calorie counting may well actually be accelerating the obesity problem. Someone who is overweight with a fat tummy is likely to be producing too much insulin or be insulin resistant, but in their quest to lose weight they are following a low-calorie diet as recommended by the FSA – and are therefore eating a lot of starch. Starch is relatively low in calories and perceived to be healthy, but the starch is causing a significant insulin release which is forcing their body to store more fat. The perfect example of this is the baked potato with cottage cheese. This would be a low-calorie option but is also one that is likely to cause a high insulin response – and someone with a fat tummy is likely to overproduce insulin after eating it.

Chasing after low-calorie options would, therefore, appear to be making some of us fatter than we need to be.

SATIETY – FEELING FULL

Perhaps one of the most memorable talks I heard in Denver was a paper on the link between feeling full (satiety) and eating protein. In my view, one of the many marvels of the world is the biochemical affect of eating protein. When you eat a lump of meat, which is predominantly protein, you are ingesting essential amino acids which contain peptides. When your body breaks up the protein in your stomach and your alimentary canal, the peptides are released and send a message to your brain to tell you that you are full.

Research has shown that one of the benefits of increasing protein levels in the diet is that the dieter feels fuller for longer.[5] It has been proven that protein makes you feel fuller for longer when compared to fat or carbohydrates (including whole-grain starch).

So we know that eating protein, as opposed to starch, will make you feel fuller for longer. This has nothing to do with calorific value, because the actual calorific value of protein tends to be lower than that of whole-grain starch, so the simple calculation of calories is misleading.

A low-calorie diet which is also low in protein will not be as satisfying as a high-protein option, and satiety (feeling full) is a useful weapon in the battle against the bulge.

SUSTAINABILITY AND PRACTICALITY

Calculating the amount of calories in foods requires either some very fancy machinery (not readily available), a book by McCance and Widdowson called *The Composition of Food*, or you could resort to a high street calorie guide which is often incomplete.

If none of these options are available you need to stick to processed foods which have been labelled by their manufacturers. This is pretty strange in a world where we are being told to eat fewer processed meals by the same calorie-counting health experts – and I am struggling to understand how we are supposed to measure the calorie content of food accurately without being dependent on supermarket ready meals.

As hunter-gatherers we did not see a passing bison and calculate the amount of calories we were about to consume. Indeed the whole notion that this is appropriate reflects a poor understanding of cooking in a kitchen, or of real sustainability. The process of calculating calories is a modern concept which forces our nation to be largely dependent on the food industry, which in itself makes the measurement unsustainable. We know the biggest issue with weight loss is sustainability and clearly this method of measuring food is generally not sustainable without dependence on food companies.

Just recently, it was also shown that some of the manufacturers have been incompetent at calculating the calorific content of the food they are producing.[6] This comes as no surprise considering the possibility for error in any manufacturing process, and again it highlights how dangerous it is to build a nutrition policy which is largely dependent on food manufacturers.

METABOLIC RATE

For me, the issue over the metabolic rate illustrates just how cunning the human body is and why the simplistic message of calorie counting from government bodies makes a mockery of science.

Humans evolved as hunter-gatherers and therefore had to survive in times of feast and famine. When food was plentiful they would eat as much as they could and when things got tough they survived by living off their fat. So our bodies are programmed to cope with feast and famine. There are natural indicators of famine and when those kick in the body will do everything it can to preserve life.

So when you reduce the amount of food you eat, the body will recognise the reduction in calories and, if this continues over an extended period, it will comparatively reduce its metabolic rate.[7] This is a perfect way to conserve energy. So eating less can, for many, mean that the body simply starts to slow down; while you are calorie counting your body is energy counting. As many experienced dieters have found out, during the first week or so you lose lots of weight on a calorie-controlled diet, but then weight loss slows down as the body slows down to accommodate the reduction in calories. This is really very annoying but inevitable.

The BNF have suggested that you may 'fool' your body out of this behaviour by feeding the body with the same weight of food but with fewer calories. They suggest that you eat lots of foods which are high in water – but as far as I am aware there is no proper randomised/clinical evidence to suggest that this is correct. This is the same sort of logic that came up with the calorie-counting concept.

Again, calorie counting may be accelerating the obesity problem by reducing the metabolic rate – and when we return to higher-calorie meals (as we always do), we regain the weight lost, and sometimes add more, as our metabolic rate has been lowered.

NUTRIENT FAMINE

Another obvious problem with measuring food by reference to calorie content is the lack of information on nutrients. Food is not just about energy. Food isn't there just to provide us with petrol; it is there to help us keep well, build cells, feed our brains and do many other things. The foods that are really good at all these other tasks are those that contain:

- ◆ Essential amino acids
- ◆ Essential fatty acids
- ◆ Essential vitamins
- ◆ Essential minerals
- ◆ Fibre.

In Table 4.2 you can see how the different foods compare by reference to 100 calories.

	Essential fatty acids	Essential amino acids	Essential vitamins and minerals	Fibre	Rating
1 boiled egg	yes	yes	yes	no	3
40g bran flakes	no	no	no	yes	2
1.5 Brazil nuts	yes	yes	yes	yes	3
1 chocolate biscuit	no	no	no	no	0
100g kidney beans	no	yes	yes	yes	3
120g new potatoes	no	no	yes	yes	2
500g spinach	no	yes	yes	yes	3
60g steak	yes	yes	yes	no	3
36 strawberries	no	no	yes	yes	2

Table 4.2 – Nutrient contents

There's no connection between the amount of calories and quality. Then, when you take a look at the individual vitamins and minerals in each of the different foods according to a portion of 100 calories it becomes even more bizarre. I have set this information out in tables in the appendix. The idea that calorie counting will tell us anything useful about the nutritional value of the food we are eating is simply nonsense.

THERMODYNAMICS
For all you science failures like me, don't miss this bit out. I was hopeless at science at school but since I first listened to Professor Feinman explain the laws of thermodynamics I have never looked back.

The whole basis of calorie counting is explained as the simple equation that if you eat (take in) 100 calories you need to burn (use up) 100 calories, otherwise you will get fat. This assumption is a simple interpretation of the first law of thermodynamics.

There are three laws that make up the laws of thermodynamics. The first law, commonly known as the law of conservation of matter, states that matter/energy cannot be created nor can it be destroyed. The quantity of matter/energy remains the same. It can change from solid to liquid, but the total amount of matter/energy in the universe remains constant.

The classic example is the burning wood analogy. If you put wood on a fire the energy in the wood gives off heat, which is now another form of energy that escapes into the atmosphere. So, similarly, we eat food containing energy and then we use that energy in being energetic. The energy does not simply disappear. So the argument for calorie counting works as follows: if you don't burn off the energy you take in, it will be stored in the form of fat.

The second law of thermodynamics is commonly known as the law of increased entropy, which is all about wastage. Let's put this into the context of the human body and eating food. If you eat a piece of food that turns to calories easily (for example, sugar and starch), your body has to do very little to make that conversion. However, protein does not convert simply into glucose and therefore your body actually has to burn calories to make the change. So you can eat the same calories and do the same actions but if you eat protein you are likely to burn more calories.[8] While the actual extra burn of calories is not great, it has been argued in one study that this burn accounted for one third of the improved performance of one set of dieters who were eating more protein.[9] This was really well explained in a paper published in *Theoretical Biology and Medical Modelling* in July 2007

PROOF

Perhaps the biggest issue is that the theory of calorie counting as a credible means of losing weight has never been properly proven, and that when compared in clinical trials to other weight-loss methods it loses out again and again.[10] There's more on this in Chapter Six. What we do know is that over five decades of observation the average weight loss is very modest, being no more than 10 kg over a year.

Summing up

We know that eating less food or eating fewer calories does not mean that you will lose weight, and in several trials eating more produced better results.

Certain components of food, like protein, make you burn more calories and keep you fuller for longer but being low or high in calories is irrelevant. It is not simply to do with eating less.

Information on calories does not tell us if the food will generate a significant release of insulin (the fat storage hormone). Insulin is directly linked to weight gain. Eating less will not necessarily stop our bodies over producing insulin. Certain foods are likely to stimulate a high insulin response.

Calorie counting doesn't tell us if the food is nutrient rich. Nutrient-rich, rather than low-calorie, food is critical for good health.

Calorie counting is essentially unsustainable unless you intend to live off pre-prepared food and then you must rely on the competence of the manufacturer.

When compared to other diets in clinical trials calorie counting does not achieve the best results.

BIG FAT LIE 2 – EAT A DIET ACCORDING TO THE EATWELL PLATE

We have been told by the government to eat a healthy diet whether we are fat or thin, and the foundations for this healthy diet are the following eight rules, or tips as they are described on the FSA website:
1. Base your meals on starchy foods
2. Eat lots of fruit and vegetables
3. Eat more fish
4. Cut down on saturated fat and sugar
5. Try to eat less salt
6. (Get active and try to be a healthy weight)
7. Drink plenty of water
8. Don't skip breakfast.

Now, anyone reading this might believe that this list of dietary advice would be based on science or, at the very least, on the known necessary nutrient intake for human life. But, as you will see, some of it is not. To begin with the actual nutrient intake requirements for human life are as follows.[11] These can be defined as 'the essentials':
1. Water
2. Amino acids (histidine, isoleucine, leucine, lysine, methionine, phenylalanine, threonine, tryptophan and valine)
3. Essential fatty acids (linoleic and a-linolenic acids)
4. Vitamins (vitamin C or ascorbic acid, vitamin A, vitamin D, vitamin E, vitamin K, thiamine, riboflavin, niacin, vitamin B6, pantothenic acid, folic acid, biotin, vitamin B12)
5. Minerals (calcium, phosphorus, magnesium, iron), the trace minerals (zinc, copper, manganese, iodine, selenium, molybdenum, chromium), electrolytes (sodium, potassium, chloride) and ultra-trace minerals.

So does the healthy eating advice of the government match the known nutritional requirements of human existence? Well, it does if you stick to the advice on eating lots of fruit, vegetables, fish and drinking lots of water while cutting down on salt. Even the message on breakfast is good. But the main message the government is to base our meals on starchy foods and cut down on saturated fat and sugar. This message on starch and fat does not correspond to what we know about our essentials for good health. Let's look at these two instructions.

ONE – 'BASE YOUR MEALS ON STARCHY FOODS'

The first direction the FSA has chosen to give us is that we should base our meals on starchy foods, and this message is repeated by the NHS and the BDA (British Diatetic Association). Here are the exact words of the BDA:

> Plan your meals / snacks around starchy foods such as bread, chapattis, breakfast cereals, potatoes, rice, noodles, oats, pasta, etc. Aim to include one food from this group at each meal time – these foods should provide the bulk of your meal.

The FSA are so supportive of starch that they explain why we should include a significant amount of starch in our diet – notwithstanding the fact that it is a food group that is low in the essentials. Here is what they write to persuade the British public to eat more starch:

> Starchy foods such as bread, cereals, rice, pasta and potatoes are a really important part of a healthy diet. Try to choose wholegrain varieties of starchy foods whenever you can.

> Starchy foods should make up about a third of the food we eat. They are a good source of energy and the main source of a range of nutrients in our diet. As well as starch, these foods contain fibre, calcium, iron and B vitamins.

> Most of us should eat more starchy foods – try to include at least one starchy food with each of your main meals. So you could start the day with a wholegrain breakfast cereal, have a sandwich for lunch, and potatoes, pasta or rice with your evening meal.

Some people think starchy foods are fattening, but gram for gram they contain less than half the calories of fat. You just need to watch the fats you add when cooking and serving these foods, because this is what increases the calorie content.

Let's run through these statements. This may appear boring but it is essential to understand the importance the FSA has placed on starch.

First, 'starchy foods are ... a really important part of a healthy diet'. Does starch or starchy food give us a significant amount of those important nutrients which are defined as essential? The answer is very simply no, it does not. Starch does not contain any significant amounts of amino acids or fatty acids and most starches, in their natural state, are low in vitamins and minerals. While they may have some fibre, the level compares poorly to other foods.

So none of the essentials are found in abundance in starch without fortification, which is when the food manufacturer (not nature) adds vitamins and minerals to the food concerned. The food industry has been adding vitamins and minerals to cereals and other foods for years to supplement people's diets because they have not been eating the right foods. Fortification was a great idea when you had a population unable to buy foods which were naturally rich in essentials, but in modern Britain this is somewhat strange. In fact, what the government is actually doing with fortification is giving the general population vitamin and mineral tablets in a different form. So far the government has not required starch companies to add amino acids and fatty acids to starch, but no doubt it will happen if they carry on.

Look at Table 4.3 which shows you the allocation of these essentials in some different starches. Just to be fair, I have picked whole-grain starches but remember that the numbers would be lower for the white starch options.

Whole grain starch	Essential amino acids	Essential fatty acids	Essential vitamins	Essential minerals	Fibre content
Brown pasta	Low	Low	Medium (fortified with B vitamins)	Medium (high in selenium and magnesium)	Medium
Potatoes with skin	Low	Low	Medium (higher in B vitamins)	Medium (high in potassium and magnesium)	Medium (only if the skin is eaten otherwise it is low)
Brown rice	Low	Low	Medium (only if fortified)	Medium	Medium
Bran flakes	Medium	Low	High (because of fortification)	Medium (is heavily fortified with iron)	High
Wheat flakes	Low	Low	High (if fortified)	Medium	High
Brown bread	Low (does contain a source of some of the amino acids)	Low	High (because of fortification)	High	High

Table 4.3 – Essentials in some starchy foods

It is easy to see how starch, even the whole-grain version, is not full of essential dietary elements. Now let's have a look at some other non-starch foods that are rich in essentials:

Food	Essential amino acids	Essential fatty acids	Essential vitamins	Essential minerals	Fibre content
Eggs	High	High	High	High	Low
Strawberries	Low	Low	High	High	Medium
Salmon	High	High	High	High	Low
Dark chocolate	Medium	Low	Medium	High	Low
Brazil nuts	Medium	Medium	High	High	High
Spinach	Low	Low	High	High	High

Table 4.4 – Essentials in some non-starchy foods

Wouldn't it be more suitable to have a bowl of strawberries and a handful of nuts or two eggs for breakfast than any amount of starch? The eggs would keep you full for longer (remember the comparison between the satiety response of starch and protein), and the nuts with the strawberries would beat the starch hands down when it comes to fibre, minerals, vitamins, amino acids and fatty acids if you didn't add in fortification. Have another look at the tables setting out the levels of vitamins and minerals in various foods to remind yourself of the poor quality of bran and other starches.

So on the face of it it is really hard to understand the logic for saying that 'Starchy foods such as bread, cereals, rice, pasta and potatoes are a really important part of a healthy diet.'

Let's just get this clear. The government wants you to ensure that starch is 'a third of the food you eat'. So the government is keen that we get a lot of fortified starch instead of other foods which are naturally rich in the essentials.

The government also goes on to confirm that starch is great because it is 'a good source of energy'. This is fundamentally correct, and even better than just being a good source of energy, starch is a very efficient source of energy. Unlike protein which turns to energy slowly and requires energy to break it down, starch turns to energy quickly and efficiently. Efficient, fast energy is fantastic if you intend to run a marathon or do a fifteen-hour day in the fields but how many of us are doing that? What is even more bizarre about this statement is that by the government's own logic the obesity problem is to do with an imbalance between the amount of energy we consume and the amount of energy we spend. It is therefore quite illogical to want to encourage a nation that is getting fatter due to excess energy intake to eat more starch which is, after sugar, the fastest and most efficient source of energy available to man.

So we have been told to ensure that at least one third of our plate is made up of starch because it is a great source of energy and 'the main source of a range of nutrients in our diet'. We know that what nutrients there are in starch are mainly added by the food manufacturers. For people who don't eat foods like fruit and vegetables, then modern fortified cereals and starch may well be the main source of nutrients – but this, even by the government's standards, can not be a good thing. Remember they want to increase our intake of vegetables and fruit. Of course, if you follow the government guidelines it may well be true that most of your nutrients are coming from starch even though other foods would be a much better source. Fortification doesn't just mislead the public; it puts our health and welfare back in the hands of manufacturers rather than in our own control once again.

As if this was not enough we are then told that – notwithstanding the fact that we are being told to eat low-nutrient, efficient-energy foods in abundance (at least one third of our plate) – we should 'eat more starchy foods...'

The more starch we eat, the more efficient energy we will take in – which means, according to the logic of calorie counting, the more exercise we must do. We know that the nutrient level of starch is poor compared with other foods, so why on earth would you want people to eat more of this food unless they needed it to provide energy for a heavy manual job or a marathon run? Quite clearly, however, the government have some concerns over this message on starch as they do make the following statement: 'Some people think starchy foods are fattening, but gram for gram they contain less than half the calories of fat.'

If you believed that simple calorie counting was a sensible method of helping you slim this would make sense, but there are serious issues with the measurement of calories as a means of helping you lose weight, especially when you consider the impact of insulin.

There are many experts who think that starchy foods are fattening and some of these people are recognised obesity experts in the UK. These experts don't just think starch is fattening for some people; they know it is fattening. To really understand why, we need to adjourn the debate and extend our knowledge of basic biochemistry.

THE METABOLISM OF STARCH

When we eat foods rich in starch, our bodies break it down into glucose molecules in the body and absorb them into the bloodstream. Starch (whether brown or white, whole grain or otherwise) is relatively high in calorific value (i.e. rich in energy) but, as we have seen, is low in the essentials unless the manufacturer has added them. The main purpose of starch is to provide energy.

Starch begins turning into glucose as soon as it enters the mouth when saliva breaks the complex carbohydrate molecules into simple sugars. Therefore, quite soon after you eat starch there is a rise in your blood glucose levels. This will cause an increased entry of glucose into the pancreas which triggers the release of insulin. Have another look at the illustration earlier in this chapter.

As we know, insulin is very important for helping us to use glucose for energy but the body will, if we have too much glucose, convert most of the excess into fat once the liver's storage capacity is full. Some experts have discriminated between brown and white starch on the basis that the fibre in brown starch will slow the entry of the glucose into the bloodstream. These experts have argued that all that matters is the speed that food turns to glucose, because it is the glucose that stimulates insulin. The method of measuring the speed at which food turns to sugar through digestion is called the glycaemic index or GI for short. This does seem logical because we know that one of the key triggers for insulin release is the level of glucose in the bloodstream, so it would appear sensible to link insulin release with the glycaemic index of foods.

However, while this may appear very logical and sensible it is superficial and in one particular trial it was shown that GI and insulin release are not linked.[12] A perfect practical example of the superficiality of the GI index is fructose, because fructose is low GI but does stimulate insulin quite vigorously without raising blood-sugar levels. Insulin can be triggered by many physical events.

Another example showing the weakness of the simple GI argument is the case of people who suffer from the overproduction of insulin, whether or not they are actually insulin resistant. Someone overproducing insulin could eat a low-GI diet but still have a massive insulin response and start gaining fat. It is the amount of insulin in the body and not glucose that is the real indicator of whether or not you may gain fat.

In fact, we release insulin even before we start eating – just by the smell of certain foods. When we see or smell food, gastrointestinal hormones are released that will stimulate the pancreas to release a small amount of insulin. This is an anticipatory mechanism, designed to modulate any sudden influxes of glucose into the plasma or bloodstream. So the famous saying of all failed dieters – 'I just look at cake and get fat' – may not be so silly.

Fortunately there is an insulin index that shows what the average insulin response will be to different foods, but this is only an average measurement and doesn't explain what will happen to an individual who may be over producing insulin or actually insulin resistant. Basically insulin is really only triggered in any significant amounts by starch and sugar.[13] While sugar and starch are carbohydrates there are many foods in this group that do not trigger insulin, in any significant amounts, including nuts, seeds and green vegetables. If you mix protein with starch or sugar, or fats with starch or sugar, then the insulin response will go up again.

So some experts in the UK argue that:
◆ Insulin is the hormone that makes the body collect fat
◆ If you eat lots of foods that require insulin you may over produce insulin and that can lead to insulin resistance and eventually diabetes
◆ The foods that trigger insulin are primarily starch and sugar
◆ People who over produce insulin or are insulin resistant are more than likely to gain fat, particularly around the tummy
◆ The incidence of fat tummies is growing at an exponential rate and a large tummy is a key indicator of several other health problems.

Starch and sugar are making many of us fat because of the virtuous circle between the production of insulin and the conversion process, triggered by the release of insulin, of glucose to fat.

The bizarre thing is that other experts who are 'in love' with starch, like Diabetes UK and the FSA, and who recommend a high-starch diet (one third of the plate) do acknowledge that weight around the waist can be linked to type 2 diabetes, an illness linked to overproduction of insulin. At what point did they not pick up on the fact that insulin is triggered by starch?

The experts who are sceptical of the starch consumption message, as promoted by the government, are also concerned that insulin is at the root of a lot of modern health problems. The general description used is called IGF, insulin-like growth factors.

One of the key questions being asked by these experts is why there is such a close association between obesity and cancer. At the moment the biggest cause of cancer after smoking is obesity, but no one knows quite why this should be. Some insulin experts believe that with a better knowledge of insulin they can unlock the mystery. Before I refer to the actual studies the very basic thinking is as follows:

◆ There is an association between elevated insulin levels and insulin-like growth factors (IGF), long-chain proteins produced by the body that are necessary for tissue growth

◆ While insulin levels may fluctuate , IGF change more slowly. Constant highs and lows in insulin levels are likely to cause an increased level of IGF which, unlike insulin, will effectively stay at a high level

◆ Research since the 1990s has suggested that IGF plays a role in tumour progression by accerlerating the delivery of food to these hungry cancerous cells

◆ Cancer cells must have glucose to survive and grow (more about this later, in Chapter 7)

◆ Elevated levels of insulin may also be altering the levels of other hormones in the body which are distorting our natural biochemistry.

Quite a few studies have been carried out looking at the possible link between insulin and cancer. In summer 2009, there was a study published in the *International Journal of Cancer* which looked at the development of cancer and different diets.[14] The study was carried over seventeen years and included 61,000 women, and its conclusion was that diets which triggered higher levels of insulin seemed to increase the risk of breast cancer. In 2008 there was another significant study which appeared to show a link between insulin and breast cancer.[15] This study looked specifically at insulin levels in more than 800 women with breast cancer and a similar number without the disease. Women (who were not on hormone replacement therapy) with the highest insulin levels were found to be at two-and-a-half times greater risk of developing breast cancer.

These studies do not prove that heightened levels of insulin cause cancer, but they do show an association which needs further investigation urgently as most women with breast cancer are told to eat a low-fat, high-starch diet. Another 2008 study is of equal interest because here the researchers were interested in finding a connection between size and weight and breast cancer.[16] In this study those with an increased waist circumference were found to have a 35–36% increased risk of breast cancer if they were eating a diet which stimulated insulin. Other cancers have also been the subject of much research, and in 2009 a small study looking at men with prostate cancer saw a radical improvement in the containment of the cancer when the subjects were put on a low starch/low sugar diet.[17] The assumption, therefore, is that by reducing the need for insulin you can reduce your risk of cancer, and when you actually have cancer you can slow the growth of tumours.

Summing up

Without fortification, starch is not rich in the essentials, so it is not necessary for a truly healthy diet.

Starch is, after sugar, the best form of efficient energy so why would you want to feed a passive population a diet based on efficient energy?

Starch, like sugar, stimulates insulin and insulin triggers fat collection.

At present, 40% of the population are overweight with an increasing number becoming obese and developing type 2 diabetes – a disease based on the over production of insulin.

Fat tummies are becoming more prevalent at an exponential rate and fat tummies are a key indicator of over production of insulin and insulin resistance.

Insulin resistance and IGF may well be the missing link between obesity and cancer as well as other health issues.

The statement by the FSA that starch is a good source of vitamins and minerals is highly misleading.

The statement by the FSA that we should eat more starch makes no sense in the current obesity epidemic, since the FSA says we need to cut back on our energy intake. Starch is the most efficient source of energy after sugar.

Overeating of starch is in part causing the obesity crisis.

TWO – 'CUT DOWN ON SATURATED FAT AND SUGAR'

The second big message by the government is to cut back on fat and sugar. Let's look at them separately.

EAT LESS SUGAR

It is interesting that the government sees sugar as so clearly separate from starch. As we now know, starch starts to break down into sugar as soon as it enters the mouth, as saliva turns complex sugar molecules into more simple molecules called disaccarides. Once the disaccarides enter the small intestine they will be broken down into sugar. In the case of some starches the speed at which the food turns to glucose in the bloodstream will be the same as for table sugar.

So the sugar message is at real odds with the message about starch. No doubt the experts at the FSA will try and argue that starch has nutritional and fibre benefits which do not apply to sugar but, as we know, this argument is somewhat dubious . You may want to look back at the tables at the beginning of this chapter. If we removed the fortification process from starch production the argument in favour of the health benefits of starch would be nonsense. As for fibre, we know there is more fibre in green beans than there is in starch, so let's not overexcite ourselves with fibre and starch.

You may be pleased to know, however, that we are all doing what we are told and cutting back on sugar which has been reflected in the figures released by Tate and Lyle and their justification for their investment in Splenda®. Hurrah, we are doing what we are supposed to – but are we getting thinner?

EAT LESS SATURATED FAT

The 'eat less saturated fat' message is now part of our culture. The average person is said to be trying to reduce saturated fats, and we know from the food industry that the increase in products with reduced levels of saturated fats is one of the fastest growing areas for food development and production. Everyone is doing it.

Most people also believe that the fear of saturated fat is based on robust science. I attended a Unilever debate on saturated fats in 2008 which aimed to see how many people understood the messaging on saturated fats; over 90% of those taking part said that they understood the message and believed it to be correct. Good news for food manufacturers who produce low-fat food and things like butter substitutes.

The simple message being promoted by the government is:
◆ Saturated fats are high in calories and therefore are making us fat
◆ Saturated fats cause heart disease.

So do saturated fats make us fat because they are high in calories, and do they cause heart disease?

DO SATURATED FATS MAKE US FAT?

If you accept that simple calorie counting may be a little dodgy as a means of managing or losing weight, the issue over calories is irrelevant. If you accept that the release of insulin is critical to fat collection, then the most interesting piece of information you may want is whether saturated fats cause a significant release of insulin. The answer to this is simple. No, saturated fats do not cause a significant rise in insulin release when you eat the fat without sugar and starch.[18] The reason why Dr Atkins and others saw saturated fats as a useful ingredient in the fight against obesity was because saturated fats are filling and satisfying and don't trigger insulin release, especially when you eat the fat with protein. This does explain to some extent why certain tribes across the world can eat a large amount of saturated fat and not become fat. The key issue is that they eat saturated fat without also having a diet rich in starch and sugar.[19]

When studies have been done with high saturated-fat levels combined with low levels of starch and sugar, the subjects not only lost weight faster than the low-calorie, low-fat option but – even more interestingly – the cholesterol profile of the subjects on the high fat diet was better.[20]

DO SATURATED FATS CAUSE HEART DISEASE?
To even begin to try and answer this question we need to understand the history of how the link between saturated fat and heart disease became gospel. Ancel Keys, a professor in the US in the 1950s, was the first to argue an apparent link between saturated fats and cardiovascular disease. The research that he published was epidemiological in nature.

A quick lesson in the science of epidemiology:

For those who think epidemiology sounds like an unpleasant disease, it's actually a discipline in science that looks at connections and makes reasoned assumptions about cause and effect from those connections. An epidemiological study is a statistically based study and assumes likely outcomes following certain events. It does this by looking at a series of events or symptoms in a target group of people. So, for example, if you did a study of all drivers and non-drivers in the UK you might find that the percentage of drivers that is overweight is higher than the percentage of non-drivers. If there was a significant difference in the percentage of overweight people between the two groups an epidemiological study would be likely to conclude that driving increases the risk of making you fat. Clearly this is nonsense – unless you then carried out a clinical trial showing that driving makes you fat, but this would not be an epidemiological study.

Historically, epidemiological studies have been proven to be very effective when understanding infectious diseases but it is a far more complex issue to try and uncover the cause of chronic illnesses like heart disease or obesity. There are simply too many factors that could influence the outcome.

A large epidemiological study carried out into heart disease in Europe called The European Cardiovascular Disease (CVD) Statistics 2005 suggests all types of connections.[21] One could make numerous assumptions but, like all studies of this type, it covers all kinds of lifestyle issues such as smoking, diet, physical activity and alcohol. An epidemiological study does not prove cause and effect but it does suggest that there may be a connection, and it is for clinical trials to then test whether or not that conclusion is actually correct.

Unfortunately some people think that reaching a conclusion in an epidemiological study is as good as proving the point. This is not a very safe approach to science, and a really good example of an epidemiological study out of control was in relation to hormone replacement therapy in the US. The science writer, Gary Taubes, summed it up brilliantly in his book, *Good Calories, Bad Calories*: 'Poor epidemiological evidence has been described as "disastrous inadequacy of lesser evidence" when you build a health campaign without proper randomized clinical trials to substantiate the assumption.'

A recent example of the possible difference between an epidemiological study and a subsequent clinical trial is the ongoing Early Bird Study, looking at childhood obesity and exercise. Because there have been numerous epidemiological studies linking childhood obesity to a lack of exercise, a proper clinical trial was started in Plymouth to look at whether these studies were correct in their assumptions. The answer, very simply, is no. That's right – when a study was done in a controlled environment with the standards required of a clinical trial there was shown to be no cause and effect between children exercising and obesity. But more on this later.

In short, epidemiological studies are a little like hearsay in a court of law. It may be relevant to helping you build your case but it is not considered good evidence in a courtroom and will be dismissed by a judge if presented by either side.

> While this may seem very academic, it is really important to keep this knowledge in mind when you come to look at the evidence suggesting that saturated fats are killing us or making us fat. In fact you should always be a little sceptical of epidemiological studies on anything complex with multiple factors or influences.

So, back to the history of saturated fat and the heart disease gospel. Ancel Keys carried out epidemiological studies. He compared different diets and health profiles of people around the world. His original work covered twenty-two countries but he chose only six for publication in 1953. The Six Country Study concluded that there was a definite link between the intake of saturated fat and the incidence of heart disease. What is not well known is that if he had added in the data from the other sixteen countries the connection and association between heart disease death rates and fat intake would have fallen away. However, unfortunately for us, the apparent link was adopted by several influential people and the idea took hold.

In 1956 Keys published a second report called the *Seven Countries Study* which also confirmed the findings of his first study in 1953. His conclusions were that from this study he could show that:

◆ Cholesterol levels predict heart disease risk
◆ The amount of saturated fat in the diet predicts cholesterol levels and heart disease
◆ Monounsaturated fats protect against heart disease.

Since 1956, there has just been an unrelenting wave of studies trying to prove this connection. Fortunes have been spent by the food industry and others looking to find this link. The whole low-fat food industry is a product of this assumption and many brands are only worth millions of pounds because of this belief. Why else would anyone replace natural, simple butter with a highly processed and unnatural spread?

By the time the 1980s were upon us, we had a consensus of opinion based on epidemiological studies that the connection between saturated fats and heart disease was sufficiently compelling to start issuing dietary guidelines. At this stage there had not been any large scale randomised clinical trials clearly pointing the finger at saturated fat. However, one study really turned the saturated fat–heart disease hypothesis into gospel.

In 1984, the Lipid Research Clinics Study (LRC) was published. This was a study looking at cholesterol-lowering drugs and the incidence of heart attacks, published in the *Journal of the American Medical Association*. While it showed some benefits from cholesterol-lowering drugs, it was assumed by the researchers that the outcome would also be the same if people ate less saturated fats. Please note that the study did not involve saturated fats and the subjects on the trial were all middle-aged men with extremely high cholesterol levels. The test was just to look at cholesterol-lowering drugs. The assumption made by the researchers was that if you eat a diet low in cholesterol, then that would have the same effect as cholesterol-lowering drugs. While this assumption was not tested in the trial it did not stop them concluding that 'it is now indisputable that lowering cholesterol with diet and drugs can actually cut the risk of developing heart disease and having a heart attack'.

This conclusion triggered various agencies in the US to start a campaign to lower the amount of saturated fats in our diet. Indeed, if you went back and reviewed the original guidelines of the study it was clear that the trial was to test the performance of a drug. Everyone in the study was on a diet and therefore, at no time, did this study look at the effect of saturated fats on heart attacks or heart disease. So, on the basis of a study looking at drugs lowering cholesterol among men with high cholesterol levels, we ended up with a message to eat less saturated fat. Have I missed something here? Big assumptions were made.

Since the LRC study there have been twenty-six studies[22] trying to show this absolute link between the intake of saturated fats and heart disease, but of these only four show any association and those were epidemiological (those come at the end of the note for ease of reference).

Now we all know that eggs are fine but for years they were put on the 'don't eat' list because it was thought that their high cholesterol levels would cause heart disease – but thanks to the Egg Board spending a huge amount of money on clinical trials it has been shown that eating eggs in abundance does not cause your cholesterol level to rise.

It's funny how the anti-fat brigade will get very excited about epidemiological studies showing an apparent connection between saturated fat and heart disease, but fail to take account of epidemiological studies which show the opposite. In the European Cardiovascular Disease (CVD) Statistics 2005 there is some really interesting data which suggests that eating loads of saturated fat is positively good for us. This has been called the French Paradox, and Table 4.5 contains information taken from that report.

Countries	% of death rates from CHD	% of energy from fat	% from saturated fats	% of population that do no exercise in a week
France	0.2	39	15.5	52
Germany	0.3	39	13.7	30
UK	0.6	39	13.5	45
Netherlands	0.2	36	14.6	9
Azerbaijan	1.0	16	5.7	No info available
Turkey	0.2	24	7	No info available
Ukraine	1.0	25	7.6	No info available

Table 4.5 – Fat in the diet, exercise and death rates

So we know that it's not black and white, and while the French chomp away on large quantities of saturated fat doing little or no exercise (and smoking to boot), they have a low rate of death from coronary heart disease (CHD). Maybe the issue is beer (i.e. sugar) rather than fat!

There have also been another twenty non-epidemiological studies[23] which tried to show a link between the intake of saturated fats and CHD. Only six found a slight benefit from reducing saturated fats and those had many other variables from medication or supplements, or other factors such as smoking and exercise which could have distorted the outcomes.

The very best studies to prove cause and effect are called double-blind studies. These ensure that neither the researchers nor the participants know who is and who is not receiving intervention. To date there have only been two relevant double-blind studies and neither showed a connection between saturated fats and heart disease.[24]

This plea for sanity is not a lone cry. Several very influential experts such as C.A. Corr (Consultant Cardiologist Guys and St Thomas' Hospital) and and M.F. Oliver (National Heart and Lung Institute) have asked those in power to stop propagating an unproven message.

It does seem strange to find such certainty in the mind of the FSA among the pile of published science which is not conclusive in its findings. And, of course, you need to remember that for every published paper or study there will be another pile of research which is basically dumped because the outcome of the trial does not meet the preferred conclusion of the funder. A great deal of research is funded by large corporations which have a vested interested in the outcome of the study.

Against all this anti-saturated-fat evidence, there are some statistics showing quite the contrary, especially when mixed with a low-starch and low-sugar diet. A randomised controlled dietary trial published in the *Journal of the American Medical Association* in 2006 looked at the impact of a low-fat dietary pattern and the risk of cardiovascular disease in women.[25] It raised some really interesting results. Apart from questioning the whole heart health–saturated fat theory, it actually concluded that a relatively higher intake of both protein and fat can have benefits independent of weight loss on the features of metabolic syndrome which contribute to heart disease. The report on this study went on to state:

One must consider whether the dietary goals themselves,
particularly the substitution of carbohydrate for fat, were

appropriate... Indeed, the clinical trials showing cardiovascular disease benefit that have been invoked as supporting reductions in saturated fat achieved those reductions primarily by substituting polyunsaturated fat rather than reducing total fat... Overall there is little evidence that reducing saturated fat per se, without substituting polyunsaturated fat, has a direct benefit on clinical cardiovascular events.

In a study published in 2004[26] the conclusion reached was even more surprising because it showed that for post-menopausal women a diet high in saturated fats actually decreased the risk of coronary heart disease. This came as a surprise to the researchers.

Another study looked at diets and any association with ovarian or breast cancer.[27] In this particular study, the women eating a meat-and-saturated-fat diet had a 26% reduced risk of developing breast cancer. So saturated fats in this study seem to reduce the risk of cancer. We also know that saturated fats are possibly the best fuel for the heart.[28]

In one meta-analysis study (i.e. a study which reviews other studies to look for common outcomes) which looked at twenty-seven individual studies on the link between fats and heart disease no link could be found.[29] And, just to hammer home the fact that this subject is not quite as black and white as the FSA would like us to believe, the largest study on lifestyle factors and heart disease was published in the *Lancet* in 2004 and did not list saturated fat.[30]

What we really need are more clinical studies looking at saturated fat in our diet with and without the effect of starch and sugar. But unfortunately the world of health is now so obsessed with the fear of saturated fats that it won't even let us carry out clinical trials. In 2004, I asked a well-known research body in the UK to carry out a randomised clinical trial into saturated fats (different types) combined with a high- and a low-starch diet but was turned away with the explanation that they would not get ethical approval and no one wanted to know more about saturated fats anyway. I thought research was to ask questions and not presume.

So that is how it is: a hypothesis started in the 1950s which has been backed by somewhat inconclusive science and subsequently supported by people who thought it all sounded good and helpful. Nothing evil, but nothing scientifically robust. So while all our experts point at lard and suet (albeit without any particularly convincing evidence) the obesity epidemic rages on.

What is even more concerning is the fact that while some of us are getting fatter and fatter we are eating less sugar and saturated fat. It is clear from the Dietary and Nutritional Survey in 1986/87 that there has been a significant reduction in saturated fat in food for men and women.[31] Table 4.6 was taken from that report – published by the FSA!

Type of Fat	Men 1986/7	Men 2002	Women 1986/7	Women 2002
Saturated	16.5	13.4	17	13.2

Table 4.6 – Saturated fat intake

You do wonder why the epidemiologists at the FSA, and there are a lot of them, haven't bothered to read their own report in any detail. You may also wonder why, at the time that we are reducing saturated fat intake, we have the acceleration in obesity rates. We also know that the food industry is producing more and more low-fat products due to the demand created by the government instructions.[32] At the same time we also know from the FSA report that the amount of saturated fat in meat is also being reduced.[33]

Decade	% saturated fat in beef	% saturated fat in pork	% saturated fat in lamb
1950s–1970s	25	30	31
1990s	20	20	26
2007	5	4	8

Table 4.7 – Saturated fat content in meat

Am I missing something here? I am sure that the official answer would be that it is all the saturated fats found in other foods such as dairy or fast food, but that does not take away from Table 4.7 showing an overall reduction in saturated fats. Could someone, somewhere, at the FSA start to read and question their own information?

Putting aside all this wonderful information and data, there is still the argument that as humans we are designed to eat meat. From our hunter-gatherer roots, it does seem strange that we have evolved to eat a natural food which could kill us. On the contrary, it would be fair to assume that there should be benefits in the food we are evolved to eat. There is virtually no history of heart disease among the Inuit tribes who live off saturated fats with little or no fresh vegetables, and this example does not stand alone. Many hunter-gatherer tribes have diets rich in saturated fats and yet have no history of heart disease. The message telling us to strive towards decreasing fat in our diet is certainly dubious and last year (2009) a study published in the *Journal of Clinical Lipidology* showed that actually eating a low fat diet increased your risk of CHD. And anyone with A-level biology will remember that saturated fat is a key component of a group of substances called phospholipids, which are critical to building cell walls. Saturated fat plays a crucial role in the integrity of our cells.

Summing up

Sugar and starch are closely related. If sugar is not good for us I fail to see how starch, once you strip out the fortification, is so great especially when we are feeding a passive population.

There has never been a published peer-reviewed randomised clinical study which actually really shows a clear and certain link between saturated fats and heart disease without the influence of other significant factors.

We are eating less saturated fat and less sugar, and yet we are continuing to get fatter.

Our naturally evolved diet includes some saturated fats, so it does seem a little strange that these should be inherently bad for us especially for people not eating a great deal of starch and sugar.

The FSA wants us to choose starch instead of fat, but it is the starch that is making some of us fatter due to the impact of insulin and our lipid (fat) metabolism.

Saturated fats are critical for our good health

BIG FAT LIE 3 – GET ACTIVE AND EXERCISE MORE

If you could be bothered to read the NHS report, 'Statistics on Obesity, Physical Activity and Diet: England, 2006, 2008 and 2009' you would find it clear that the NHS has reached a brick wall with its obesity solution. This report states clearly that we are eating less than ever but some of us are getting fatter and fatter, faster and faster.

The epidemiologists and everyone else have concluded that the problem is exercise. They have found a correlation between thin people and exercise and have therefore concluded that thin people are thin because they exercise. But, as I have already shown, epidemiology does not test things in a proper clinical way. This means that this conclusion can only ever be a hypothesis that still needs to be tested. For example, it is also easy to conclude that thin people are thin because of their biological state, which makes them burn calories efficiently and want to do more exercise after eating. Some thin people are simply designed to be lean by their biological state.

Is it possible that exercise as a solution to obesity may be a red herring?

I began to understand this properly when I attended the European Obesity Conference in 2005/2006 at which Sir Neville Rigby spoke. At that time he was chairman of the European Obesity Task Force and was addressing an impressive audience of senior representatives from the food giants from Unilever through to MacDonald's, PepsiCo and Kellogg's. His appeal was for an understanding of the limited impact of exercise on weight loss and that exercise will not, nor cannot, ever be a solution for weight loss. Diet is the beginning, the middle and the end. At that time large food companies were trying to solve the obesity problem by contributing to the provision of sports facilities in several European countries. One could be cynical and suggest that these efforts were in order to pacify the legislators in Brussels and reduce the food legislation restricting their profitability...

Sir Neville referred to several large-scale European studies showing categorically that exercise had no significant impact on the weight management of the participants. One of the studies since that conference which has added fuel to the doubters' fire is the Early Bird Study.[34] This lost its financial support from the government because it showed that exercise made no difference to the weight loss of children. Even the most significant study linking exercise to weight loss, known as the Finnish Study 2000, suggests that the relationship between exercise and weight is more complex than had been imagined or expected.[35] Studies that have tried to prove the link between exercise and weight loss have only been able to show a 'modest affect on weight loss without dieting'. In a significant study carried out by the World Health Organisation into the obesity problem in the US it was concluded that exercise is not a factor of any influence.[36]

But there are really obvious reasons why the simplistic message of 'do more' is nonsense.

CALORIE BURN
The UK government has suggested that to stop further weight gain and help reduce weight people need to do about sixty to ninety minutes of light exercise a day. For example, swimming sixty lengths in an hour would

get through 333 calories. A cycle ride lasting an hour (assuming you are not Lance Armstrong) will amount to only 300 calories; not a lot for a pretty long session. Then you must not forget to subtract the calories you would burn anyway just by being alive which amounts to about two to three a minute – so in reality the net calorie burn is not that 300 calories, but around 150 instead. As you can see, the actual calorie burn is not that great, so you really do need to do a significant amount of exercise to make a real difference. The average person with children and a job will, realistically, struggle to fit in this amount of exercise every day. A little bit here and there is really not enough to make any real difference to weight loss, especially if you are on a starch-rich diet.

HUNGER

When you exercise, your muscle tissue – which is working hard – will draw on fat supplies to provide energy. Once you stop exercising the body will naturally wish to replace the energy taken from the fat cells that had just supplied all that energy to the muscles. This process is carried out by a combination of insulin release and the enzyme called lipoprotein lipase (LPL). This is all part of the body's natural survival mechanism, evolved over thousands of years. The more energy you expend by using up fat supplies, the more your body wants to replenish the fat after the exercise is over. To replace the fat, the body triggers hunger and sends you off searching for food. Your body is not stupid. The foods your body will crave are those that can provide efficient calories to replace its fat stocks rapidly. So most people eat starch after exercise because starch provides the fastest, most efficient energy source after sugar.

Insulin is also back in the picture again. Insulin is triggered to move energy from fat to the muscle tissue. Then it will be triggered again to replace the missing energy and, as we already know, insulin kicks in when you eat sugar and starch and the body will get back to converting glucose to fat. There have been some studies which have tried to link exercise with improved appetite regulation, but in reality there has never been any conclusive evidence of this proposal.

STRESS

If you are pretty fit anyway, your body is well adapted to exercise, but if you are obese or overweight your body may feel under stress when exercising. This has a further metabolic affect – you release the hormone cortisol, which in turn triggers insulin. So even when you are trying to do all the right things, your body could be doing something that undermines all your hard work. A study published in the *Journal of Applied Physiology* in 2003 showed that there was a release of cortisol during stressful exercise.[37] A further and very interesting report in *Hypertension*, a publication of the American Heart Association, showed the link between stress and obesity.[38] This report highlighted the tendency of obese subjects to gain weight around their stomach areas (which was similar in stressed primates) that is triggered by glucocorticoid secretion. What was noted in that report was that levels of cortisol in normal men were lower than in obese men.

Ultimately, there is fundamentally insufficient robust evidence that exercise will have a significant impact on weight or inch loss. At the same time there is an argument that asking obese patients to exercise (unless it is very gentle exercise) could be counterproductive because it causes a hormonal response which actively makes the body collect and cling on to fat.

EXERCISE AND HEALTH

While this book may question the logic of doing exercise to lose weight, there is no doubt that exercise is an excellent tool for weight maintenance and is fantastic for our general health.

The message that exercise is good for us is great and should be shouted out loud – but what is really misleading for a great many people is the idea that exercise will significantly help them lose weight. As we know, we may eat less but our metabolic rate will reduce accordingly, and then we'll do more and, guess what, we'll eat more!

The exercise that can help with weight loss is anaerobic exercise rather than aerobic exercise. Anaerobic exercise helps build muscle and the more muscle mass you develop the higher your metabolic rate will be, therefore the more fat you can burn for energy. Unfortunately most people become obsessed with burning calories and evaluate the exercise by the calorie burn rather than the whole metabolic process.

So say no to beasting (a term used by the fitness profession) and let's be honest with those who are significantly overweight – eat a different diet and go to the gym when you have lost the weight through diet because without doubt regular aerobic exercise can help you maintain weight once you have reached your target size.

Summing up

Exercise has never been shown to really have a massive effect on weight loss.

Making people do lots of exercise in the hope of losing fat is misleading in the extreme.

In some cases anything other than gentle exercise can actually cause weight gain.

Exercise can make you eat more.

Ship of fools

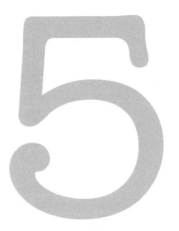

Recently I was asked a really interesting question about the Data Protection Act. My inclination was to answer the question immediately; after all, I have several qualifications in law and been paid a small fortune to provide legal advice. However, I held my tongue and gave the name of another lawyer in a data protection practice. It would cost more than free advice from Hannah Sutter but at least the answer would be guaranteed to be right.

The person who had asked me the data protection question had already taken advice from a lawyer in general practice in her local town of Bournemouth and, while he meant well and had been confident in his knowledge, he was wrong; simple as that. What we learn from this everyday issue is that subjects like law are immensely complex and the title 'lawyer' does not mean that someone knows everything about the law. A great tax lawyer will be fantastic at sorting out a difficult tax problem but you would not want that tax lawyer negotiating your divorce or advising you on a criminal offence.

Biochemistry and human physiology are really no different from law in this respect. Biochemistry and physiology are huge topics and cover a vast amount of information and knowledge, all of which is constantly changing. Someone who is an expert in hormones would not necessarily know a great deal about inborn errors in metabolism. The key thing in all big disciplines is to know when to say 'I don't know but I know someone that does'.

This might well seem irrelevant but at the moment the eatwell plate is presented by the FSA as the absolute rule on what we should and should not eat. Everyone is relying on it as the 'right diet' and every day articles

are written by journalists which refer to the eatwell plate. The journalists are not alone, as all the following expert bodies follow the eatwell plate guideline:
- ◆ Diabetes UK
- ◆ British Nutrition Foundation
- ◆ The NHS
- ◆ British Dietetic Association.

So who are the people behind the FSA website and the eatwell plate? Who are the people responsible for making some of us fatter than we need be? Are they best qualified to pass comment on what we should and should not be eating or are we going to find that we are effectively taking advice from the wrong people? In other words, am I asking the tax lawyer a question I should ask of a criminal lawyer?

The actual FSA has a board made up of the following individuals who are ultimately responsible for the website content. They are:
- ◆ Jeff Rooker
- ◆ Dr Ian Reynolds
- ◆ Professor Graeme Millar
- ◆ John W. Spence
- ◆ Professor Maureen Edmondson
- ◆ Professor Sue Atkinson CBE
- ◆ Tim Bennett
- ◆ Margaret Gilmore
- ◆ Clive Grundy
- ◆ Michael Parker
- ◆ Chris Pomfret
- ◆ Nancy Robson
- ◆ Dr David Cameron.

These individuals have sought out other experts to advise them on certain aspects of the web site content and in particular there is the Scientific Advisory Committee on Nutrition (SACN). This has replaced the original committee called COMA (Committee on Medical Aspects of Food Nutrition and Policy).

So here are the individuals who sit on SACN and who advise the board, which no doubt relies on what they have been told:

◆ Professor Peter Aggett (interest in trace element metabolism in health and disease)
◆ Professor Annie Anderson (special interest in cancer and nutrition)
◆ Professor Sheila Bingham (interest in cancer and diet)
◆ Mrs Christine Gratus (expert in advertising and marketing)
◆ Dr Paul Heggarty (expert on nutrition and genes)
◆ Professor Alan Jackson (nutrition and foetal development)
◆ Professor Timothy Key (studied veterinary medicine nutrition and epidemiology – interests are roles of diet and sex hormones in the aetiology of cancer)
◆ Professor Peter Kapelman (interest in diabetes care and obesity)
◆ Professor Ian MacDonald (special interest in obesity)
◆ Dr David Mela (Unilever)
◆ Dr Ann Prentice (nutritional aspects of bone health and osteoporosis)
◆ Dr Anita Thomas (interest in thrombosis)
◆ Mrs Stella Walsh (consumer expert)
◆ Dr Anthony Williams (child nutrition).

How could these recognised experts be so wrong?

REASON 1 – WRONG EXPERTS

This is an impressive list of names, but when you look closely at their areas of expertise only one is an expert in diabetes and only one has a special interest in obesity. The rest are a mixture of experts in various discrete aspects of nutrition, epidemiologists, well-meaning members of the public with no real expertise in nutrition and, guess what, a representative of Unilever.

All these people are well-intentioned, highly educated individuals, but again it is like going to the best tax lawyer when you've been charged with murder. I can assure you that a tax lawyer would be clever and very brilliant at what they did but they won't know about or be interested in your murder case.

The FSA Committee has also various subcommittees which are entrusted with certain specific areas of interest. These subcommittees are called working groups:
◆ The Approaches to the Nutritional Assessment of Novel Foods Subgroup
◆ The Energy Requirements Working Group
◆ The Folate/Cancer Working Group
◆ The Iron Working Group
◆ The Subgroup on Maternal and Child Nutrition
◆ The Carbohydrate Working Group.

The Carbohydrate Working Group is relatively recent (it was set up in 2008) and is designed to look at carbohydrates within these terms of reference:

To provide clarification of the relationship between dietary carbohydrate and health and make public health recommendations. To achieve this they need to review:
◆ The evidence for a role of dietary carbohydrate in colorectal health in adults (including colorectal cancer, IBS, constipation), infancy and childhood
◆ The evidence on dietary carbohydrate and cardio-metabolic health (including cardiovascular disease, insulin resistance, glycaemic response and obesity)
◆ The evidence in respect to dental health that has arisen since the COMA report 'Dietary Sugars and Human Disease' (Department of Health, 1989)
◆ The terminology classification and definitions of types of carbohydrates in the diet.

Now look at the experts on this key committee. You might expect, as I did, that it would be full of biochemists and endocrinologists (experts in hormones, including insulin) with a special interest in carbohydrate metabolism. Well, it isn't.

The experts chosen to sit on this committee are :

◆ Professor Ian MacDonald (metabolic physiology)
◆ Professor Alan Jackson (nutritionist)
◆ Dr David Mela (Unilever)
◆ Professor Timothy Key (epidemiologist with a special interest in cancer)
◆ Professor Anne Anderson (food choice expert)
◆ Mrs Christina Gratus (ex-advertising executive).

Have I missed something here? The terms of reference are, without doubt, based on scientific evaluation so I am at a loss to understand what Professor Anne Anderson and Mrs Christina Gratus have to add to the debate.

Let's take an even closer look at these individuals, especially Alan Jackson and Professor Ian MacDonald who are probably the nearest thing to the correct experts.

Here is the detail on Ian Macdonald:

Ian Macdonald is Professor of Metabolic Physiology at the University of Nottingham and Director of Research in the Faculty of Medicine and Health Sciences. His research interests are concerned with the nutritional and metabolic aspects of obesity, diabetes and cardiovascular disease, with additional interests in nutrition and metabolism in exercise. His research involves studies in healthy subjects and various patient groups, and combines whole body physiological measurements, molecular investigation of tissue samples, and dietary interventions. Ian Macdonald is presently President of the Nutrition Society, Editor to the International Journal of Obesity and Chair of the International Association for the Study of Obesity Finance Committee.

Very impressive stuff, but surely what we need is someone who can really get to grips with the affect of insulin on our bodies?

Now for Alan Jackson:

> Alan Jackson is Professor of Human Nutrition, School of Medicine at the University of Southampton. Professor Jackson's current work explores the extent to which modest differences in maternal diet and metabolic competence influence foetal development, predisposing to chronic disease in adulthood. Professor Jackson was a member of the Committee on Medical Aspects of Food and Nutrition Policy (COMA) for ten years and was a Consultant Adviser to the Chief Medical Officer on Nutrition from 1989 to 2002. Professor Jackson is a member of the EFSA Panel on Dietetic Products, Nutrition and Allergies.

Another very impressive CV, but again I don't see any special interest in carbohydrates and insulin. You will note that this chap was a member of COMA which was first responsible for the eatwell plate. I hardly think he has much of an interest in the impact of insulin on human metabolism and fat gain.

So there we have it. A wonderful group of very highly qualified experts but no one who has a real focus on carbohydrate metabolism.

REASON 2 – FEAR OF FAT

Another reason for the composition of the eatwell plate may well be a misplaced fear of fat and, possibly, protein. We known that the nutritional benefits of starch are poor (see Chapter 4) so I can only assume that it is fear of fat and protein that makes the FSA emphasise the importance of starch.

It was in 2007 that I first became suspicious of the messages from the FSA. I asked for reports supporting the reduction of saturated fats in our diet and I was sent by the FSA 'Independent Advice on Possible Reductions for Saturated Fat in Products that Contribute to Consumer Intake', by Geoff Talbot, known as the fat consultant. This document is really a practical guide on how you persuade food companies to change their products to comply with the proposed new guidelines. The FSA also sent me a report entitled 'Scientific Review of the Microbiological Risks Associated with Reductions in Fat and Added Sugar in Foods'. This was really a technical analysis of the shelf life and quality of foods with lower levels of sugar and fats.

What I then asked for was the evidence on which the FSA had decided to go ahead and recommend a reduction in our saturated fat intake. I was referred back to the references at the end of the report put together by Geoff Talbot. He is a chemist with a special interest in the manufacture and production of fats. The report he had prepared was to support the pressure on the food industry to develop products that would fit the new criteria. However, having been a sad lawyer, I decided to work my way through the ten pages of references to seek out the robust evidence proving categorically that saturated fats were causing cardiovascular disease (CVD), etc.

Seventeen hours of excruciating boredom later, I did not find any robust evidence that saturated fat causes heart disease but I did find references to papers arguing that there was no link between saturated fats and heart disease – for example, 'The Low Fat/Low Cholesterol Diet Is Ineffective' from the *European Heart Journal* of 1997. This categorically confirmed that 'the commonly held belief that the best diet for the prevention of coronary heart disease is a low-saturated-fat, low-cholesterol diet is not supported by the available evidence from clinical trials'.

Is it not remarkable that a document provided by the government to support the reduction of saturated fats is actually quoting a significant review telling us that there is no link between saturated fats and CVD? Perhaps there is a real need for a proper subcommittee on fats just to be sure that they actually know what they are publishing.

A perfect example of fat fear getting in the way of good sense is the egg fiasco. For several years we were told by the FSA that eggs were really bad for us because they were high in cholesterol, and this was assumed to cause high cholesterol levels in people who ate them. In 2009 the

University of Surrey finally finished off the campaign against eggs with their study that allowed the British Heart Foundation and others to change their position on them. Did you know that for about ten years before this several experts repeatedly said that eggs were fine?

Fear based on robust science is fine, but perhaps it is now time for the FSA to set up a subcommittee on fats to really get to grips with the information out there.

REASON 3 – UNDUE INFLUENCE

We know that a representative of Unilever sits on the main committee of the FSA, so perhaps the long arm of corporate influence is clouding the issues. This may sound slightly far-fetched, but you need to ask questions because promoting starch in the UK today with the health problems we have does not make any sense. Remember, only thirty years ago the tobacco companies did everything they could to stop the link between cigarettes and cancer being publicised. Fortunately employers, with the support of lawyers, took hold of the evidence and stopped the nonsense through the law courts. Yes, it was the lawyers and employers who actually created the comparatively smoke-free world that we now live in, something most people are thankful for.

The starch and sugar companies are some of the largest companies in the world by a long way. For instance Kraft turns over approximately $50 billion yearly and PepsiCo's revenues for last year were $45 billion with Kellogg's trailing along with just $12 billion. These companies have a vested interest in selling us high-starch products. This is how they make their money, and boy do they make money: for example, Kellogg's operating profit for 2009 was in the region of $2 billion. This is very relevant because we know that most research produced in the Western world is ultimately funded directly and indirectly by large corporations in the ultimate pursuit of profit. The research that supports the high-fibre or low-fat message has been heavily funded by industry and not by government. To take one instance, go and have a look at the companies that make contributions to Diabetes UK which then provides funding for research. The connection between the advancement of science and corporate interests is unavoidable but it could be one of the main reasons why much hard work and research has simply been ignored. When the Atkins diet took off in the early part of 2000/2001, its success was reflected in the diminishing sales of pasta and fruit juice in the US. In fact two large corporations blamed their insolvencies on the low-starch, low-sugar message. Within twelve months of these events, the food industry responded by emphasising the idea of a low-GI option, spearheaded by many, including Tesco. The fantastic thing about the low-GI message is that you can still keep selling the starch and sugar message but you highlight the whole-grain or fructose version. How wonderful – sell more starch and sugar under the health message of low GI. But we know how misleading 'low GI' can be to what is actually happening in your body. The main problem for the no-sugar, no-starch message is that the only winners in the story are the vegetable and meat farmers and all the big companies that currently dominate our food industry would be put out of business. There simply hasn't been effective lobbying and investment in research by the meat marketing board or the fruit and vegetable growers' association. Even if they wanted to invest in research they don't have the funds because the profit on non processed fish, meat, diary and vegetables is poor.

Now let's look at the various interests of some of the people who sit on these key committees...

Member	Personal interests		Non-personal interest		Any other interest
	Company	Nature of interest	Company	Nature of interest	
Professor Alan Jackson	None	N/A	Nutricia Clinical Care Baxter Healthcare	Sponsors of Annual Nutrition Course	None
Professor Peter Aggett	None	N/A	School Activities Astra-Zeneca Nestrec ILSI Wellcome Yakult Individual: New Zealand Dairy Goat Council Cadbury Schweppes	1–8. Chairmanship (meetings) and lecture fees Departmental research and education in medicine and health, including food safety and metabolism Consultancy: Research Project Management Consultancy	None
Professor Annie Anderson	None	N/A	None	N/A	None
Professor Sheila Bingham	None	N/A	None	N/A	None
Mrs Christine Gratus	None	N/A	None	N/A	None

Member	Personal interests		Non-personal interest		Any other interest
	Company	Nature of interest	Company	Nature of interest	
Dr Paul Haggarty	Smith Nephew Diageo Café Direct	Shareholder Shareholder Shareholder	Pharmaton Editorial Consultant on the American College of Physicians' Information and Education Resource. Editorial Consultant on the Nutrition & Health conference and German Society for Reproductive Medicine	Unpaid advisor on pregnancy study protocol Consultation fee contributed to research funds Lecture fees contributed to research funds	None
Professor Timothy Key	None	N/A	None	N/A	Member of Vegetarian Society of the UK Member of Vegan Society
Professor Peter Kopelman	Weight Watchers International	Medical Adviser	Alizyme Pharmaceuticals	Clinical trial sponsor	Member of Governing Board – Institute of Food Research Scientific Adviser, Foresight, Department of Innovation, Universities & Skills

Table 5.1 – Scientific Advisory Committee on Nutrition – main committee, declaration of interests (continues overleaf).

Member	Personal interests		Non-personal interest		Any other interest
	Company	Nature of Interest	Company	Nature of Interest	
Professor Ian Macdonald	Mars Europe CocaCola Europe	Advisory Board European Scientific Advisory Committee	Mars Incorporated/ Mars Europe Unilever Nestle	Research project funding; PhD student funding Research project funding; PhD student funding Research project	Board member, Obesity International Trading (trading company owned by International Association for the Study of Obesity)
Dr David Mela	Unilever	Employee and shareholder	None	N/A	None
Dr Anita Thomas	None	N/A	None	N/A	None
Mrs Stella Walsh	None	N/A	None	N/A	Consumer representation for National Federation of Consumers FSA and DEFRA Committees and working parties, including Cattle Movement, and Food Borne Disease
Dr Anthony Williams	None	N/A	None	N/A	Trustee, Women and Children First Fellow, UNICEF (UK)

Member	Personal interests		Non-personal interest		Any other interest
	Company	Nature of Interest	Company	Nature of Interest	
Dr Ann Prentice	The Biosciences Federation	Honorary Officer/Director	As Director of MRC Human Nutrition Research responsibility for institutional interests as listed:		
			BBC	Consultancy	
			Institute of Brewing & Distilling	Research Funding	
			Mars Ltd	Consultancy	
			National Association of British and Irish Millers	Consultancy	
			Optimal Performance Limited	Research Funding	
			Tanita UK Ltd	Research Funding	
			The Coca Cola Company	Advisory Board	
			The Beverage Institute for Health and Wellness	Research Funding	
			Weight Watchers International Inc	Research Funding	

Table 5.1 – (Continued)

As you can see, some of our experts have strong connections with large food companies that really benefit from selling lots of foods full of sugar and starch.

REASON 4 – IGNORANCE OR INNOCENCE

This is probably the toughest argument. There is no doubt that the sheer quantity of publications providing information on diet each day, each week, each month, is enormous. Perhaps these guys have simply not got round to reading the papers published on insulin and carbohydrate intake.

REASON 5 – PREJUDICE

One of the most irritating aspects of lawyers is the fact that they don't agree with anything they have been told until they have satisfied themselves that it makes sense, which is why the law of this country has developed by case law and constant changes to judgements. Lawyer after lawyer challenges the assumptions of the lawyers who came before them. Our very training at law school and at degree level is based on questioning everything, even if it is a judgement by a law lord. Law evolves because, as a profession, lawyers say 'Yes, *but...*' This training is not always common in other subjects and I wonder whether the lack of questioning of what appears to be a certainty is one of the main reasons we are held back from solving the obesity crisis today.

Frequently lawyers are instructed to go over old ground on a matter that might seemed closed to re-evaluate the evidence or judgements passed. So nothing is sacrosanct and nothing is presumed. Because of this training lawyers have learned to accept that judgements can change and that someone found guilty of murder may be innocent and vice versa. Lawyers don't have a problem with changing their minds, especially if knowledge becames available which undermines the previous decision. It would seem that science and scientists do not always deal with change or new evidence so easily.

This difference in training was really apparent when I recently recruited a young nutritionist to join the team at golower. She was bright and able and had good qualifications. While she was keen to take the job she was slightly concerned about our position on starch. We gave her the job because every single person who comes out of university today with a degree in nutrition is certain that whole-grain starch is good and saturated fats should be reduced to a minimum.

When I asked how she knew that whole-grain starch was good and saturated fat was bad she referred, very confidently, to the lectures she had attended and the textbooks used on her course. I then asked for the science – the published, clinical science which proves these two facts. At this point the young nutritionist was slightly confused. To put her out of her misery I presented her with some of the studies referred to in this book, all of which were published in peer reviewed journals, which show how low-starch diets (with and without saturated fats) make people thinner and healthier more quickly than normal low-fat, low-calorie options. Within four weeks the nutritionist concerned was asking a whole heap of good questions about some of the assumptions that she had been taught at degree level as being fact.

We are all burdened with what we have been taught, and it is hard to sometimes walk away from what appears to be a certainty, especially if you have written the nation's diet on the back of some seemingly unreliable evidence.

TURN THE SHIP AROUND

What we do know is that there is a significant body of clinical evidence showing that a diet low in starch and sugar will help reverse the weight and related health issues of obese and overweight people and people who are diabetic or pre-diabetic.[1] How long can it be right to ignore the evidence? At what point do we need to question the experts who are holding the evidence back from the general public? This feels a little like the *Titanic*; can someone please see the icebergs?

As this ship cruises towards disaster, I am reminded of the law of negligence and the associated duty of care. This duty is at the forefront of any ship's captain as he steers his ship towards its goal which, in this case, is a healthy and slim nation. If you keep hitting icebergs but continue to sail your ship towards them regardless of the weather and sea conditions, it would be considered a breach of a duty of care. While I am not suggesting legal action in this book I am amazed that no one in the FSA is questioning the guidelines they are busy handing out.

As the good ship UK sails towards diabetes and obesity in unprecedented numbers, notwithstanding the improving exercise levels and reduced calorie consumption on deck, it is the duty of the captain to ask whether the route he has chosen is best suited for the weather conditions he has come across. If a board of directors of a company carried on with a policy which was clearly not working they would be sacked. If you went to your GP for medicine that made you worse you would change your doctor or complain. What you don't do is keep doing what is not working.

Naturally I would expect the FSA to tell us that either we are not doing what they have told us to do properly or that we just need to wait to see the obesity number improve. Hello? We know from commercial and government statistics that we are doing what we are told. We are eating less saturated fats. We are eating less sugar. We are eating less fat. We are eating less. We are doing more exercise. We are eating more starch. We are eating more fruit and vegetables. A poor tradesman always blames his tools.

So what could we do at the FSA to improve the dietary advice given out?

First and foremost, anything to do with health and diet needs to be based on robust science and not on apparent links, however compelling. So let's not rely so heavily on epidemiologists. Second, let's get some experts in endocrinology and pure biochemists who have an interest in diabetes and obesity. You might find that the focus moves from fear of fats to concern over starch.

Then we should remove all corporate representatives on any government committee (and perhaps we need to understand why there are ex-advertisers sitting on specialist carbohydrate or other nutrition committees). Finally, we should also stop the idea that one diet suits all. This is the same as saying that one type of medicine suits all.

Summing up

The FSA is relying on expert advice which may not be appropriate for sorting the obesity crisis.

We need appropriate experts at the FSA who understand insulin and other hormones and their effect on our metabolism.

There needs to be a subcommittee on fats to investigate the effect of different fats on our metabolism, with or without starch and sugar.

We need to think about alternative eatwell plates for different people with different issues.

We need to come clean with the public and tell them that starch is not essential for human life and that most of its nutritional benefits are added by industrialised fortification.

We need to stop doing what is not working.

Let's get back to our roots

6

Those of us who are getting fatter and fatter are either not doing what we are told (although the evidence suggests otherwise) or the advice is not working. Where is the solution? Is it in the hands of the bariatric surgeon or in the wallets of the large pharmaceutical companies with their fabulous drugs, or shall we just carry on doing what we have been doing for the past thirty years unsuccessfully? Do we keep pointing the *Titanic* at the icebergs hoping that we can patch things up with the help of medics, or could we do something different which is based as much on science as possible?

To understand what we can do it is really helpful to go back to what we evolved to eat, because the laws of evolution tell us without any doubt that this will be the most perfect diet for humans – unless you don't agree with Darwin.

OUR NATURAL DIET HISTORY

Modern humans or *Homo sapiens* are thought to have first appeared about 140,000 to 110,000 years ago. Before this point there were several evolutionary changes that took us from ape to man, which are summarised in Table 6.1 on page 82.

Our evolution has been away from a quasi-vegetarian diet to one which was dependent on meat or fish, which allowed the brain to develop and which in turn was critical to our ascendance. We know that there was a move away from vegetation by the remains showing a diminishing size of the jaw, and the finding of rocks used for the butchering of animals.

Type	Years ago	Diet	Key body development features	Benefit	Evidence
Hominids	6 million years ago	Similar to chimpanzees (insects, eggs and fruit vegetation)	Smaller canine teeth/larger molar teeth allowing chewing of roots, etc	Broader food choices, all year round	Remains showing similarities to chimpanzees
Homo habilis	2.5 million years ago	Similar to hominids	Bigger brain (but still only half the size of *Homo sapiens*)	Use basic stone tools	Meat remains and cranial changes
Homo erectus	1.7 million years ago	Stronger reliance on meat because of colder climates with less vegetation. The world is generally cooling	Taller, stockier, bigger brains	Migration into colder climates	Wear on teeth remains indicate heavy meat diet. Butchering of meat evident. Development of fire. Reduced jaw size as vegetation in diet reduced
Homo sapiens	140,000 years ago	Omnivores	Even bigger brains	Best diet for survival	Development of stone age tools

Table 6.1 – Evolutionary changes

For the vegetarian sceptics, meat and associated fats are essential for building brains. More animal fat in the diet meant not only additional energy but also a source of ready-formed long-chain polyunsaturated fatty acids (PUFAs) including three key fatty acids which together make up over 90% of the long-chain PUFAs found in the brain grey matter of all mammalian species.[1] Marrow is high in arachidonic acid which is key to building brain tissue, as is docosahexaenoic acid which is also found in brain tissue itself. Suddenly cannibals don't seem so stupid![2]

As our brains grew as a result of eating meat, we were able to come up with novel ideas like the use of fire, which in turn gave us greater choices as well as improved nutrition. There can be no doubt that the discovery of the deliberate use of fire was critical for our development as it allowed us to eat a broader range of foods and improved our chances of survival.

This is a very, very short summary of our nutrition history, but it is important to appreciate our journey from ape to man as it explains to some extent how we became dominant. As the rules of evolution apply brutally, whether we like it or not, our success was fundamentally based on eating meat and fish.

Today there are still some hunter-gatherer tribes and their diet certainly helps us to understand our own diet history better. A comprehensive study of hunter-gatherer diets was published ten years ago in the *American Journal of Clinical Nutrition* which analysed the diets of many modern hunter-gatherer populations around the world.[3] The authors broke down the tribes by reference to their environment and analysed their diet by reference to calories from each food source. There's a summary of the research in Table 6.2.

Environment	% from plants	% from hunted animal foods	% from fished animal foods
Tundra, northern	6–15	36–45	46–55
Northern forests	16–25	26–35	46–55
Temperate forests, mountainous	36–45	16–25	36–45
Desert grasslands	46–55	36–45	6–15
Temperate grasslands	26–35	56–65	6–15
Subtropical bush	36–45	26–35	26–35
Subtropical forest	36–45	46–55	6–15
Tropical grassland	46–55	26–35	16–25
Monsoon forest	36–45	26–35	26–35
Tropical rainforest	26–35	26–35	36–45

Table 6.2 – Hunter-gatherer diet by environment and food source

Nearly three-quarters of all the people analysed lived on a diet based on over 50% of animal foods. Only 13% relied on vegetation for more than half of their diet, and 20% of the hunter-gatherer tribes were either solely or nearly entirely dependent on hunted or fished animal foods. Almost no tribes were solely or nearly entirely dependent on vegetation. The dependence on animal food rises the further you get away from the equator.

So we know from contemporary hunter-gatherer tribes that meat and fish are key elements of our natural diet. At what point did we start thinking that a meal should be based on starch rather than meat or fish?

About 10,000 years ago humans began to switch their food source from wild collection to basic agriculture. This change was still taking place 2000 years ago in some parts of the world. In human history this is a recent event; remember, for 130,000 years most of us were basing our meals on protein.

The hunter-gatherer life is often regarded as brutish and hard but the real facts of the matter show a very different story. While it would be fair to say that a young hunter-gatherer may have had a high chance of a violent death from a wild beast,[4] from skeletons found in Greece and Turkey we can see that hunter-gatherers were taller than their farming descendants by a good 16–17 cm. Notwithstanding the benefits of modern science and health care, the modern Greeks or Turks are not as tall as their hunter-gatherer forefathers.[5] We know from tooth enamel remains that the hunter-gatherers were not suffering from malnutrition and iron deficiency anaemia, unlike their farming descendants. A study of skeletons dating from early Neolithic times to 1500 BC found that people became increasingly prone to disease at the time farming was introduced.[6]

But none of this should come as a surprise. Just looking at the nutrient content of starch in Chapter 4 shows the paucity of essential nutrients in this food. Is it any surprise that the health and well-being of the hunter-gatherer was far greater than that of the farmer? Wheat, rice and corn – which form the basis of most Western diets – are deficient in certain vitamins, minerals, amino acids and fatty acids essential for human life, but a diet based on protein and some fruit and leafy vegetables certainly wouldn't be. Even levels of fibre are quite different between hunter-gatherers and their farm-working descendants. Fibre in rice and wheat is predominantly insoluble while that from fruits and vegetables is mainly soluble and, therefore, while the total fibre intake was probably similar the actual overall effect would have been quite different.[7]

So our diet began to change about 10,000 years ago, and slowly but surely this change has spread across the world. The initial benefits of this change, years ago, are not hard to see; the ability to create high- and fast-energy food (albeit poor in nutrients) was compelling for many. With agriculture there came many social changes, setting in play our development towards industrialisation. Naturally, over a long period of time and with the advent of modern medicine and public health policies, our general health has improved. What is most evident is the natural marriage between efficient-energy crops and intensive labour.

The idea that hunter-gatherers had to work hard to get their food is a fanciful notion not based on any robust evidence. Studies of the few remaining hunter-gatherer societies show that these people work less hard than their farming neighbours while enjoying healthier lives. So where does this all take us? We moved to a starch-based diet at the same time as we moved to a labour-based lifestyle – for the majority, that is. This labour-based lifestyle has continued for many people throughout the world in different ways. While we had an industrial revolution, it did not diminish the need for cheap labour: workers who required cheap food to provide cheap, efficient energy in order to carry out their labours for low salaries. Starch is without doubt the best form of food for labourers, especially if you don't really care about their nutrient intake or the length of their useful lives. Having nutrient-rich food for the mass population has only been a recent feature of Western society.

From the end of the 1950s, Western society began to change again as we moved into a post-industrial era and away from labour-based industries – the start of the move from mechanical production lines to computers. Slowly but surely we have became less dependent on sweat and tears for the expansion of our economies, and digital power has taken over.[8] The US started this move in the 1950s and we began the same journey about ten years later. It has been said that 'production is shifting from material goods to information processing activities, fundamentally changing the structure of these societies'.[9]

Just look at Table 6.3, which shows the swing away from manual labour towards office work in the UK.

% of working population	1951	1961	1971	1981	1991	2001
High professional	1.8	2.6	3.3	4.1	4.9	5.1
Lower professional	4.6	6.2	7.9	10.9	12.6	14.6
Employers and owners, managers and administrators	10.6	12.2	13.2	15.6	20.8	21.2
Clerical and secretarial	11.1	13.5	14.8	15.6	14.9	13.9
Skilled manual	23.4	22.1	19.7	16.4	13.8	10.9
Semi-skilled manual	31.3	28.4	26.2	24.7	22.8	23.8
Low-skilled manual	17.2	15.1	15.0	12.7	11.2	10.4

Table 6.3 – Changing patterns of work in the UK, 1951–2001.[10]

The number of people doing professional or management jobs has gone up from 17% to almost 41% and, at the same time, the low manual percentage has drifted from 71% to 45.1%. This reflects a massive swing away from physically intensive labour.

But let's see what has happened in the last few years. All those dramatic changes have slowed down and really the big changes took place in the 1970s and 1980s. Table 6.4 looks at more recent figures.

% of working population	2001	2006
High professional	5.1	5.8
Lower professional	14.9	16.4
Employers and owners, managers and administrators	21.2	22.0
Clerical and secretarial	13.9	12.3
Skilled manual	10.9	10.3
Semi-skilled manual	24.4	24.0
Low-skilled manual	10.4	10.3

Table 6.4 – Changing patterns of work in the UK, 2001–2006

What is clear is that we have become a very different society since the end of the industrial period and the cut off point, if any, is probably the end of the 1970s, into the early 1980s.

This is not intended to be a book on social change, but it is inevitable that as we become less reliant on labour there should be changes in what we eat. When people do eight or more hours a day on a factory floor or are involved in manual labour in the fields or elsewhere, it would be perfect to fuel the human engine with starch – especially if you don't really care whether the workers' diet is rich in nutrients. But if you want your workers to sit still and think or use their fingers, ears and tongues rather than their biceps then a diet based on starch has to be a little foolish, since the key message with starch is that it is energy efficient. Without the benefits of industrialised fortification it is really poor in the essentials.

As we know from other chapters, if the average person eats starch and then doesn't do something extraordinarily energetic the excess energy, in the form of glucose, will be quickly transported to the liver and either stored as glycogen or converted to fat. There are two solutions to this problem. Either change how we work and live or change what we eat.

Changing how we work is not possible. We can't go back to the pre-modernisation, pre-computer era which kicked off about fifty years ago. In the face of these work changes the government is desperately trying to change how we live by encouraging exercise, but as we know from Chapter 4 we would need to do masses of exercise to make any difference to the amount of starch we are consuming and make any in-roads in to the obesity problem. The other alternative is to think about what we eat. Is starch right for the foundation of a modern diet where we are sitting all day, even with the sixty-minute trip to the gym five times a week?

Probably the question that our experts need to ask themselves is 'Why eat a pre-industrial diet in a post-modern society?'

Whichever way you look at the facts, the eatwell plate may suit the diet of Britain in the 1950s, but sixty years later it looks unbelievably foolish and reflects a deep misunderstanding about the role of starch in the history of the human diet. We know that starch is poor in the essentials for human life without industrialised fortification and we know that humans can live very well without starch, so why push starch down our throats when our lives today do not require the only natural attribute of starch – instant or efficient energy? For those of us lucky enough not to have a tendency to overproduce insulin a diet rich in starch is probably not an issue, but for those who are overproducing insulin or are insulin resistant starch is really not a great foundation for a healthy diet.

At the same time we know that our evolutionary success has been in part down to a diet rich in meat and fish. So it seems even more strange to have an eatwell plate which only dedicates two-fifteenths to meat and fish – very low for such an important ingredient in our natural diet.

THE REAL SUPERFOOD DIET

The hunter-gatherer diet is the diet we evolved to eat and dates back millions of years. The basic diet of hunter-gatherers from the northern hemisphere would include:

◆ Red meat
◆ Poultry
◆ Organ meats
◆ Fish
◆ Green leafy vegetables
◆ Berries and other seasonal fruit such as apples and pears
◆ Nuts and seeds
◆ Eggs.

You will notice that there is no starch listed.

Today many of these foods are described by nutritionists as 'superfoods' as they offer high nutritional value with many different benefits. Let's just review the benefits of these different foods.

RED MEAT
This is packed with high-quality protein, with most meats providing the nine essential amino acids, and it offers a high source of iron. Red meat is also a nutrient-dense source of zinc and phosphorus, both required for growth, development and maintaining the immune system. It is also an abundant source of vitamin B12, niacin and vitamin B6 which help to release energy from food. It is much easier for the body to absorb the phosphorus content in red meat than that present in cereal.

POULTRY
Chicken is extremely high in protein. In particular, it is high in the essential amino acid tryptophan (which converts to serotonin in the body). Chicken also contains high amounts of vitamins B3 and B6, and minerals such as selenium and phosphorus.

ORGAN MEATS
These are high in iron and zinc as well as vitamin B12 and folate. They also contain a high amount of vitamin A; in fact, liver is the only meat that contains a significant amount of vitamin A. Organ meats are also abundant in the minerals copper and selenium.

FISH
Fish is another extremely good source of protein, containing an abundance of essential amino acids. It also contains a high amount of vitamin D and selenium. All fish, in particular oily fish, has a high level of omega-3 fatty acids. These omega 3s can help lower your blood pressure, lower your heart rate and improve other cardiovascular risk factors such as your cholesterol profile.

GREEN LEAFY VEGETABLES

This group of foods are a rich source of minerals, especially iron, calcium, potassium and magnesium, vitamins K, C, E and many of the B vitamins, including high amounts of folate. Green leafy vegetables also contain powerful phytochemicals including beta-carotene, lutein and zeaxanthin. These substances are powerful antioxidants that help protect the body against all forms of cancer by destroying free radicals. Both lutein and zeaxanthin are also known to prevent degenerative eye diseases and cataracts. Beta-carotene is known to be important in enhancing the immune system.

Vitamin K is in high abundance in dark green vegetables, with about one cup providing around nine times the minimum recommended intake. It has become an increasingly important vitamin as it is a key regulator of blood clotting and is thought to be involved in the prevention of diseases such as osteoporosis, atherosclerosis, arthritis and diabetes.

Green leafy vegetables also provide much-needed fibre in the diet to maintain good gut health.

BERRIES AND LOCAL FRUIT

All berries are extremely high in vitamin C, and we need this vitamin to maintain a well-functioning immune system. They also contain high amounts of iron, potassium and folate as well as both soluble and insoluble fibre.

As well as providing many vitamins and minerals, berries are rich in phytochemicals and consequently in antioxidants. Anthocyanins are a group of phytochemicals that give the berries their red colour. Ellagic acid is another major phytochemical found in virtually all berries. All of the phytochemicals in berries have been shown to help inhibit the metabolic pathways which can lead to cancer. A diet rich in berries has also been shown to improve levels of HDL ('good') cholesterol and improves blood pressure levels as well. Berries also have benefits for heart and brain health. Blueberries and raspberries have the highest antioxidant capacity of any fruit.

Apples are packed full of antioxidants including quercetin, catechin, phlorizin and chlorogenic acid which all help to prevent free radicals occurring in the body and so combat oxidative damage. They are also extremely high in both soluble and insoluble fibre which has been shown to help prevent high cholesterol, while also being very high in vitamin C. Most of the apple's fibre and quercetin is contained in the skin of the fruit.

Pears are extremely high in both vitamin C and copper, and vitamin C is important for optimal immune function. They are also extremely high in fibre, with around one pear providing 15% of the body's daily value. Not only is fibre good for helping to prevent constipation, and so protect gut health, but it has also been shown to lower cholesterol levels as the fibre in the colon binds to bile salts and carries them out of the body. Bile salts are made of cholesterol and so the body must then break down more cholesterol to make more bile, and hence it reduces overall cholesterol.

NUTS AND SEEDS
Nuts are one of the best plant sources of protein. They are rich in fibre, phytonutrients and antioxidants such as vitamin E and selenium. Nuts are also high in plant sterols and are a source of omega-3 fatty acids which have been shown to lower LDL ('bad') cholesterol. Seeds contain protein, fibre and are also high in vitamin E and omega-3 fatty acids. They are also a good source of iron and zinc.

EGGS
Eggs are packed full of nutritional benefits, including vitamins A, D, E and the B vitamins, as well as containing high amounts of minerals such as iron, zinc and phosphorus. They are also very high in protein, while being one of the relatively few foods containing all the essential amino acids. Eggs are also one of the few foods that are a good source of vitamin D, an essential aid in the absorption of calcium and phosphorus. They are a good source of choline, a trace mineral required by the body for optimal brain health and which also has a major impact on cardiovascular health. Having a deficiency in choline can lead to a deficiency of the B vitamin

folic acid. Eggs contain no carbohydrates and, because they are packed with protein, they have a high satiety index and so keep you feeling fuller for longer.

Despite previous misconceptions, eating eggs does not seem to raise cholesterol levels. The yolk of the egg does contain high amounts of cholesterol but it has been shown that consuming one or two eggs a day does not have any effect on the level of cholesterol in the body.

As you can see this diet is very rich in the essentials and no fortification is required. All these foods can either be eaten raw or cooked very quickly and simply, and require no further processing.

THE REAL SUPERFOOD DIET AND HEALTH

So the hunter-gatherer diet is high in protein and low in starch and sugar. Simple as that is, and whatever the FSA may tell us, the reality is that we have evolved to eat lots of meat, fish, nuts, seeds and vegetables and not a great deal of sugar or starch.

One of the perceived negative effects of the hunter-gatherer diet is that it will have adverse effects on someone's health. However, historical and archaeological evidence has actually shown hunter-gatherers to be generally lean, fit and largely free from any signs and symptoms of chronic diseases such as CVD, diabetes and obesity which are now plaguing the twenty-first century.[11] When modern hunter-gatherers adopt a Western lifestyle, diseases such as obesity, type 2 diabetes and atherosclerosis become evident.

Let's have a quick canter through some of the issues starch lovers and promoters have raised against a hunter-gatherer diet. You must remember that if we all suddenly decided to return to a diet closely related to our evolved diet then some of the largest food companies would go out of business...

CARDIOVASCULAR DISEASE

Cardiovascular disease is fast becoming one of the main killers in the West. It includes heart attacks, strokes, high blood pressure and other illnesses of the heart and blood vessels. CVD can be caused by many things, but the main one is, of course, the diet which we follow.

At present it is recommended that we obtain less than 30% of our total energy from fat, with less than 10% coming from saturated fat. It is believed that consuming too much fat (particularly saturated fat) will cause clogging of the arteries and so lead to atherosclerotic plaques which will in turn lead to CVD. However, studies of hunter- gatherer diets have actually found that their diet would have exceeded the recommended amount – and it is suggested that they would have consumed as much as 43% of energy as fat. The evidence also indicates that hunter-gatherers were free of signs and symptoms of CVD. Perhaps a more 'up-to-date' view on this comes from the Inuit population, who consume a very high-fat diet and yet have a low incidence of coronary heart disease.[12]

It is also believed that consuming a diet high in protein and fat will also have adverse effects on a person's cholesterol profile. However, despite hunter-gatherers having a diet high in saturated fat and, consequently, cholesterol, it has been noted that their total cholesterol manifested as 'low' with levels averaging around 3.2 mmol/L.[13]

Perhaps one of the main explanations of this is to do with the high amount of omega-3 fatty acids found in the hunter-gatherer diet through the high level of ingestion of foods such as fish, nuts and seeds.[14] As well as this, it is believed that the replacement of fat with carbohydrate often results in a relative increase in plasma VLDL and triglyceride concentrations while also lowering HDL levels, indicating that basing our diet around starchy foods could actually have negative effects on the cholesterol profile.[15]

This would indicate that in fact following a diet based around that of the hunter-gatherer would actually have more positive effects on heart health and consequently decrease the incidence of CVD.

BONE PROBLEMS

At present a common public health problem is osteoporosis. Osteoporosis is a condition which affects bone, causing it to become weak and fragile to the point of breaking. The NHS has estimated that one in two women and one in five men over the age of fifty will fracture a bone as a result of osteoporosis, with approximately three million people in the UK having the disease. It is predominantly termed a female disease due to the menopause and the consequent change in oestrogen levels.

Two of the key measures to prevent developing this disease are through weight-bearing exercise and diet. The key dietary requirements to help prevent the development of this disease are through adequate consumption of calcium and vitamin D. The most recent National Diet and Nutritional Survey (NDNS) has indicated that women do consume just above the recommended nutritional intake (RNI) (n=760 mg) but around 5% of women are actually consuming below the RNI. As well as this, the main sources of calcium are milk and milk products, but around 30% is provided by cereal and cereal products through fortification. Over a third of this contribution actually comes from white bread, which of course is a starchy carbohydrate and has a very high insulin index. Obviously it is important that people (particularly women) consume adequate amounts of calcium, but should we not also be concerned about where they are getting it from?

Another major consideration related to the source of the calcium consumed is how well the body utilises it. Milk and milk products are one of the best sources, and the calcium from them can be readily absorbed. However, though vegetables and fortified foods may contain good levels of calcium, it is not as 'bioavailable' – meaning that less will be absorbed compared to the calcium from dairy products. In addition to this, plant foods contain substances like phytates which bind to calcium and so inhibit absorption. To give you an example, it has been said that about 30% of milk calcium is absorbed compared to only 5% from dark green vegetables like spinach.

Another key dietary requirement is vitamin D as it helps in the absorption of calcium. There is no set requirement for vitamin D as it can be obtained from sunlight and so it is very difficult to measure how much a person is actually getting, but there is a general consensus that people should receive around 10 µg (micrograms). The amount of foods containing vitamin D is actually pretty limited and includes egg yolks, oily fish such as herring and sardines, and fortified food (margarine has to be fortified with vitamin D by law). From the NDNS, the average intake through diet is around 3 µg; again the major source is fortified cereal and cereal products. With government guidelines recommending us to consume low-fat food where possible, it means that many individuals will consume skimmed milk rather than full-fat milk. This has implications for all the fat soluble vitamins (A, D, E and K) as they will be stripped out along with the fat, meaning that people are not getting all their essential vitamins where they are most readily found.

If osteoporosis is fast becoming a public health problem and diet can be a key preventative measure, then perhaps looking at another dietary approach such as the hunter-gatherer diet would be beneficial. It has been shown that hunter-gatherers generally maintained a greater cortical bone mass than modern humans, and so had a greater bone strength and resistance to fractures as they often developed a high peak bone mass.[16, 17]

It is often believed that high-protein diets could actually have a negative effect on bone and so increase the risk of osteoporosis, but it has been found that this is not the case. It is believed that the metabolism of dietary protein is associated with acid generation which can reduce blood pH and so cause calcium losses.[18] However, as a hunter-gatherer's diet is also abundant in fruits and vegetables, it is believed that, as these foods are alkaline, they would have buffered the high acid and so urinary calcium would be reduced.[19, 20]

METABOLIC SYNDROME

Metabolic syndrome combines many of the main health problems of the Western world including type 2 diabetes, high blood pressure, heart disease and dyslipidemia. The main cause of these disorders is a result of insulin resistance. Insulin resistance occurs when the target tissues of the body cannot respond to the standard level of insulin produced. In order to combat this the pancreas must increase its workload to produce more insulin, but eventually it will not be able to keep up with the demand and so insulin resistance will develop. This sets the scene for the progression of diabetes as the body will now have abnormally high levels of both insulin and glucose. One of the major treatments for insulin resistance can be through diet.

It has been shown that diseases of insulin resistance are rare or completely absent in hunter-gatherer diets.[21] This would indicate that their way of eating should surely be considered for the treatment of metabolic syndrome. One of the major ways in which insulin resistance develops is when someone consumes a diet which is high in refined carbohydrates and so causes a sustained level of glucose in the blood, resulting in the body needing to produce more insulin.

Refined grains such as cereals, white bread, potatoes (foods which we are advised to eat), etc., all have a very high glycaemic index/load which will cause elevations in blood-glucose concentrations. There is now substantial evidence to indicate that long-term consumption of such carbohydrates can adversely affect metabolism and health (so resulting in disorders of metabolic syndrome).[22]

As well as the glycaemic index/load of foods, the insulinemic effect of food can also be looked at in terms of the treatment of metabolic syndrome. This is particularly interesting when we take a look at fructose, a sugar found in fruit which is abundant in fruit juices. We are recommended to consume five portions of fruit and vegetables a day, with fruit juices possibly contributing to this. However, what many people do not realise is that fruits such as bananas and grapes and, in particular, fruit juice actually have as high an insulinemic effect as refined cereals – in fact, higher than doughnuts![23] This raises the question of whether fruit juices and fruits higher in sugar should be avoided by those with metabolic syndrome.

DISEASES ASSOCIATED WITH A LACK OF ANTIOXIDANTS, VITAMINS AND MINERALS

It has been well proven that the hunter-gatherer diet was vastly abundant in vitamins and minerals, and so hunter-gatherers did not experience any health concerns derived from a deficiency in any of them. A good way to document this is to look at all the disorders which can occur when hunter-gatherers deviate from their way of eating.

VITAMIN C DEFICIENCY

This was perhaps relatively unknown to this population, as their level of vitamin C was always extremely high because they ate so many fresh fruit and vegetables. However, as agriculture took over it meant that the consumption of cereal grains increased and fresh fruit and vegetable consumption decreased. Cereal grains have no vitamin C in them at all, and so high consumption of cereals will lead to a decrease in the intake of a very powerful antioxidant.

VITAMIN A DEFICIENCY

Again this would rarely have been seen in the hunter-gatherer population as they ate vast amounts of red meats, including organs such as liver as well. They also ate vast amounts of fruits and vegetables which provided excellent sources of beta-carotene which can be converted to vitamin A by the liver. The whole concern about eating a low-fat diet in today's society means that many people (particularly women) will not eat red or organ meats as they are considered too high in fat, particularly saturated fat. Vitamin A has many functions in the body such as being essential for fighting infection and disease and maintaining good eye health.

VITAMIN B DEFICIENCY

Again this would rarely have been seen in the hunter-gatherer population but it does appear to be becoming a problem in today's society. Many people believe that whole-grain cereals are rich sources of vitamin B (mainly because they have been fortified) but they are a poor source compared to lean meats, fruits and vegetables. In actual fact many whole grains can actually affect the absorption of many of the B vitamins. For example, whole-grain foods can affect the absorption of biotin in the body which can result in dry, brittle fingernails and hair. Perhaps this does not seem to be a major issue, but many people are forever trying to find a supplement to combat these types of problems, though they could all be stemming from our 'healthy eating'.

Perhaps a more extreme example of vitamin B deficiencies is the beri-beri epidemic which occurred in Japan and Southeast Asia. Beri-beri is a deficiency of thiamine. The population's main staple was brown rice but in the late 1800s polished rice was introduced, and people switched to that variety. Eventually it was discovered that the thiamine contained in brown rice was being removed in the polishing process, resulting in people not obtaining enough and developing beri-beri. This disease is rarely seen nowadays but this is only because our rice has to be fortified to include thiamine back into it. This raises the question of whether we should be eating a food if a vitamin has to be added back into it to prevent disease.

FOLATE DEFICIENCY
This type of deficiency is becoming of greater interest in pregnant women as it has been found that a lack of folate, a B vitamin, during pregnancy can cause birth defects such as spina bifida. A pregnant women is recommended to consume 400 mg/day (double the standard amount) and in order to help with this level the government has decided to enrich refined cereal grains, such as white bread, with folic acid. However folate is abundant in dark green leafy vegetables, nuts and seeds and meats, so why are women not recommended to eat these foods instead of starchy carbohydrates?

IRON DEFICIENCY
It is estimated that around 1.2 billion people have anaemia, a disorder which can occur when they do not consume enough iron, and this deficiency is more prominent in women as their recommended daily allowance (RDA) is double that of a man due to menstruation. Again, many refined carbohydrates such as cereals and white breads are fortified with minerals such as iron; however, they also contain

compounds called phytates. Phytates are a phosphorus compound which is found primarily in cereals and legumes. They bind with minerals such as iron (as well as calcium and zinc) and so interfere with their absorption by the body. Anaemia can be debilitating as it can severely affect energy levels and make people prone to a lot more infections. Hunter-gatherers would not have experienced this type of deficiency, as lean meats and animal foods are very high in iron and also have a very high bioavailability to the body, making them very easy for the body to absorb. Anaemia is perhaps one of the most preventable deficiencies of the twenty-first century, treatable by simply following the correct diet.

FURTHER EVIDENCE FOR THE PROSECUTION IN FAVOUR OF OUR REAL SUPERFOOD DIET

Hunter-gatherer diets, therefore, are effectively high in protein and low in starch and sugar. Some nutrition experts (though not any at the FSA) believe that the solution to some of our modern diseases, like diabetes and CVD, can be found in our natural diet, and that this type of diet would be better for us whether we are thin or fat.[24] This was shown in a paper published last year when people of a normal weight and size still benefited from the switch to a hunter-gatherer diet.[25] This study concluded that 'Even short-term consumption of a Palaeolithic-type [hunter-gatherer] diet improves blood pressure and glucose tolerance and decreases insulin secretion, increases insulin sensitivity and improves lipid profiles.'

But this book is about the obesity crisis and whether we are being given good advice by the government on how to deal with and solve this problem. The FSA tells us to:
◆ Eat less by reducing calorific intake
◆ Base our meals on starch
◆ Reduce our intake of saturated fats and sugar.

This is low-fat/low-calorie, high-carbohydrate fare, so what we really want to do is compare this proposal to the natural human diet (which is low in starch and sugar and high in protein) and see what results they bring in a controlled environment. This is not the world of epidemiology. This is real science.

There have been quite a few studies done in recent years following the humiliation of Atkins. but before I take you through some of them it is worth reading an extract from a letter written by Professor Broom (the founder of the first MSc course in obesity in the UK) to a another doctor interested in the validity of low-starch/sugar, high-protein diets for the management of obesity. As they say, 'straight from the horse's mouth':

Low carbohydrate diets were in fact first reported by Dr Banting in 1863 but had been used in ancient Egypt to treat 'sweet water disease', i.e. presumably type 2 diabetes mellitus. The most up to date review of the use of such therapy is in *Obesity Reviews* in an article by Hession et al.[26] This looks at a total of 1222 patients in thirteen different studies, each lasting for longer than six months. It is easy to find three-month studies but such a length of study is really inappropriate for any conclusions to be made. At six months the weighted mean difference in weight change was -4.5Kg in favour of the low-carbohydrate group (p<0.00001) although this reduced to -1.5Kg at one year (p<0.05).

Over the thirteen studies the difference in attrition rates from the studies was very highly significant (p=0.001) in favour of the low-carbohydrate approach, i.e. such an approach was more acceptable to the patients than a low-fat approach.

Cardiovascular risk parameters over the time period showed greater improvement with the low CHO approach at six months, but with little difference at a year, i.e. BP, HDL chol., triacylgycerol, with the LDL chol. demonstrating less of an atherogenic profile but not less in amount. These data are similar to others reported worldwide, e.g. Bravata et al.,[27] Brinkworth et al.[28] In addition other papers by Bravata and others have indicated marked improvement in insulin sensitivity with time in patients on low-CHO approaches.

One criticism of low-CHO/high-protein diets has been their theoretical risk of renal impairment. This relates to the high protein content of such approaches but there is no evidence to suggest diets high in protein have any adverse effect on renal function. If, however, there is already an element of renal dysfunction then high-protein diets can aggravate the problem, and as you are aware where there is a problem with renal impairment then a low-protein dietary approach is adopted by most clinicians. Clearly if the % of CHO is reduced in the diet then fat% is increased, but since the overall energy content of the diet is also reduced the absolute amount of fat is actually less than on the standard diet recommended by Diabetes UK[29].

Diets high in protein are also known to increase satiety, whereas diets low in CHO are ketogenic, and the increased level of ketone bodies leads to a reduction in appetite. Both of these effects are additive and lead to a marked reduction in food intake. Patients are therefore able to sustain for longer periods of time a much greater reduction in energy intake than on standard low-fat approaches.

Lastly, it is extremely important to realise that patients can become just as fat, if not fatter, on diets high in CHO than on high-fat diets.

Let me just run through some of the comparative studies individually. Many of these studies made headline news in the US but did not get a hearing in the UK, which is a great shame for those of us who do believe that the British public should get a choice about which way to manage their weight.

A review in 2008 considered the effects of different diets on appetite regulation, metabolic parameters, body weight and body composition.[30] The conclusions were simple:

◆ Low-carbohydrate, high-protein diets appear to be more efficacious (efficient) in lowering BMI, improving lipid (cholesterol) levels and controlling satiety (feeling full) in the short term compared to low-fat diets

◆ Increases in dietary protein may be more beneficial than carbohydrate restriction alone in terms of increasing satiety and metabolic advantage

◆ Reduced hunger through alterations in gut hormones delayed gastric emptying and improved insulin resistance

◆ Low-carbohydrate, high-protein diets may be an effective choice for weight loss, enhanced satiety and improved metabolic parameters.

In 2009 there was a further study comparing low-fat versus low-carb, high-protein diets.[31] The major findings of that study were that after initial substantial weight loss, a high-protein diet prevented weight regain and resulted in even further modest weight and body-fat loss compared with the high-carb, low-fat diet.

A significant study (which made CNN morning news) was published in 2008.[32] It compared low-fat, low-carb and Mediterranean diets and the low-carb, high-protein option resulted in a better cholesterol profile as well as better weight loss.

The year before, another comparative study was carried out in the UK looking at weight loss between the two diets using diabetics, and again the low-carb diet won on speed of weight loss and improved cholesterol profile.[33]

Another study which did not want to go the whole hog but simply looked at what happens when you reduce the amount of starch in your diet also had a positive outcome. Just by reducing the carbohydrate amount in the diet down to 130 g per day you could improve your cholesterol profile, as well as reduce weight faster than the low-calorie, low-fat option.[34] Had the participants reduced their intake of starch and sugar even further the lipid (cholesterol) profile would probably have been more impressive.

To stop boring you with more evidence let me just point you in the direction of a study published in 2008 reviewing all the comparative studies.[35] The conclusion was as we have seen above. Low-starch/sugar, high-protein diets beat low-fat, low-calorie, high-starch diets both in terms of speed of weight loss and cholesterol profile.

But losing weight is not just about actual weight loss and improving your cholesterol profile. It is also about keeping the weight off: sustainability. Again the review looked at this very issue and confirmed that low-carb, high-protein diets had a better long-term outcome.

Some organisations like Weight Watchers have taken these studies to indicate that protein is the key, but anyone who understands the studies would appreciate that the combination between high protein and low carb is what makes the diets so effective. You need the low starch and low sugar to control insulin release, and you need the high levels of protein to ensure satiety and build muscle as well as contribute towards nutrient value and calorie burn.

FEAR AND IGNORANCE OF HIGH-PROTEIN / LOW-CARB DIETS

It is possible that the FSA are just as frightened of high protein as they are of saturated fats. When Atkins took off about eight years ago, many 'experts' started to wring their hands in despair while wailing about the terrible health problems associated with low-carb diets. Most had to admit the diet worked in terms of weight loss, but they thought we were all going to die from renal failure, cardiovascular disease, bowel cancer, stomach cancer, nutrient famine...

This was no less than either bad rumour-mongering by the pro-starch brigade or simple incompetence, because until recently there were no studies looking at the side effects of a high-protein, low-carb diet. In a court of law these rantings would have been described by a judge as hearsay. Unfortunately the diet industry is not run to the same standards as a court, so you can pretty much say whatever you want and get away with it.

Since that time, however, studies have been completed looking at the possible health side effects of changing back to our natural diet away from the modern high-starch diet. There have now been several studies looking at these fears and they could find no evidence of health problems associated with low-carb, high-protein diets.[36] This issue was also covered in the Hession Study.[37]

The bowel cancer fear was based on an assumption that low carb meant low fibre. This assumption reflected a poor knowledge of nutrition and a poor understanding of what a low-carb diet actually means. We know that when it comes to fibre you are better eating nuts, seeds and green vegetables than starch, and low carb does not mean low in vegetables or low in nuts and seeds. Most of the carbs you drop in a low-carb diet are those that come from sugar and starch, neither of which is needed in order for human life to flourish.

The fear of stomach cancer and some other illnesses like renal failure was linked to the apparently high levels of meat in a low-carb, high-protein diet. We know that we are designed to eat lots of meat so the levels in a low-carb, high-protein diet are not much different to what a hunter-gatherer would eat. To add to the misunderstandings, no one seemed to notice the fact that the large-scale studies showing a link between protein/meat intake and cancer were studies which were based on the subjects eating a diet high in starch *and* high in meat. There has never been a study looking at stomach cancer and other cancers with a proper low-carb, high-protein diet. From the studies referred to at the beginning of this chapter, there are certainly experts who believe that cancer is only a problem today because of our modern diet being based on a high-starch, high-sugar combination. What we do know is that a low-carb diet may actually improve the chances of not developing cancer, due to the low-insulin effect that low-carb diets bring with them. For more on this, go back to Chapter 4.

And then there is the classic fear that poor old Atkins was buried with. We will all die of cardiovascular disease if we eat a diet high in protein and low in starch. This was based on the following assumptions:

◆ A low-carb diet is low in fibre and studies show that high fibre intake is linked to improved heart health. This is why all your cereal packets talk about whole grain. A low-carb diet (properly followed) is far from low in fibre, and in fact the fibre from nuts, seeds and green vegetables and some fruit is far better than the fibre you can get from starch and cereals.

◆ A low-carb diet is high in saturated fats. This is not necessarily so and you can choose to have a diet high in saturated fats or one that is low in them. In any event, the link between saturated fats and heart problems is not as robust as some would have you think – and remember that all the studies linking saturated fat to heart disease are working with a diet that is also high in starch.

◆ One of the key indicators of heart health is cholesterol profile. In all the comparative studies comparing low-carb to low-fat diets, the cholesterol profile of the low-carb group is better.

Just recently (September 2009) a study published in *Cardiovascular Diabetology* looked at comparative diets (low carb/high protein versus low fat) and again the low carb group has improved cardiovascular risk when compared to the low calorie, low fat group.[38] In addition the low carb group lost more weight. At one year the low carb group showed great reduction in blood pressure and waist size. They also had bigger improvements in triglycerides and HDL cholesterol at six months.

With regard to nutrient famine, I think it is pretty plain from this chapter that anyone banging on about nutrient famine should go back to the textbooks or change job. What nonsense!

If anything (apart from the FSA) has made me despair, it's the very naughty researchers who publish misleading papers. Recently a paper was published comparing low-fat to low-carb and low-calorie diets, and its conclusion was that there was no difference between the different ones.[39] In the case of the low-carb group, participants had their carbohydrate intake reduced to 200 g a day. In reality this reduction is simply not enough to make any difference to the metabolic process, and gives the impression that low-calorie and low-fat are as effective as low-carb diets. We do need a definition of low carb, because quite clearly some people are using its lack of definition to mislead the public. But more on this in the next chapter.

With all that we know about our hunter-gather forefathers, as well as those tribes still around today, together with the science that has been published, surely it is time for those in authority to accept that a pre-industrial diet (starch based) in a post-modern world is not working, and that we should go back to our roots to get a new diet for a new age. Surely we should stop the lies being written about what is and what is not good for us.

Summing up

Our evolution from ape to man involved eating a diet rich in meat without starch.

Our evolved diet (hunter-gatherer diet) is rich in all the essentials that we need in order to survive and prosper as humans. Why would we have evolved to eat a diet which is bad for us?

The hunter-gatherer diet is almost the very opposite of the eatwell plate.

We no longer live like peasants, so why feed us like peasants?

The health benefits for almost anyone who switches from a modern starch-based diet to our natural diet are compelling.

In comparative diets low-carb, high-protein diets beat low-fat, low-calorie options, both in terms of speed of weight loss but also in cholesterol profile.

Low-carb, high-protein diets have been shown to be more sustainable than low-calorie, low-fat options.

Most of the recent criticism of low-carb, high-protein diets has been based on ignorance of the nutritional make-up of the diet and a lack of evidence to support these allegations.

Ketosis – the natural obesity solution

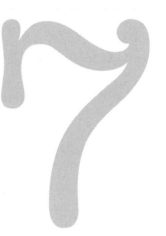

Isn't it extraordinary that we live in a world where the only solutions proffered by the health experts to deal with obesity are these?

◆ Diet – based on eat less and do more; not founded on science but sounds sensible and intuitively correct
◆ Drugs – not very effective but easy to dispense and very good for drug company profits
◆ Bariatric surgery – very expensive but can be very effective.

Each of these three options has quite obvious drawbacks. Meanwhile we are living with a natural obesity solution in our bodies: non-starvation ketosis.

Non-starvation ketosis has been scientifically proven to be very effective in weight loss and has the following benefits:

◆ It is entirely natural but not proven
◆ It does not require a prescription
◆ It does not require a surgeon
◆ Very low calorie diets are difficult to adhere to and sustain.
◆ It only requires natural, real, whole food.

Anyone can do it as everyone's bodies are designed to do it. For those unfamiliar with the word 'ketosis', it is the technical term used to describe the process of burning fat for fuel.

Humans evolved successfully to dominate the planet because we were good at eating all kinds of food and surviving in all kinds of conditions and, in particular, we had the ability to deal with famine as well as feast. To survive famine you must be able to collect and store food when there is plenty, and while you and I might use the freezer or the larder, in the good old days when we roamed the planet nomadically we had only the body for storage.

Our bodies are well designed for us to eat as much as we can and store any excess to use later. In fact, it would not be unreasonable to suggest that anyone who is obese today is a true descendant of our evolutionary forefathers. The ability to gain fat is a key to surviving a famine. Before the advent of the freezer or larder, we would naturally burn our body fat to keep us going through a famine. This is really a very clever feature of our bodies; we are naturally designed to collect fat and then use it to survive.

So how does ketosis occur, and why should it be considered a suitable tool in the obesity battle?

There are only three ways for a body to go into ketosis. You need to starve yourself by eating less than 520 calories a day, doing some extreme exercise or depriving your body of instant energy in the form of sugar and starch. In all circumstances the body will switch to burning its own fat to provide energy. To convert excess fat into energy the liver increases its production of ketone bodies which come from fat to replace glucose. This is not ketoacidosis, which is quite different.[1]

To activate ketosis without starvation or giving up your day job to spend all your time in the gym, the level of starch and sugar in the diet needs to be very low, about 60 g or less a day. Any diet that is higher will struggle to trigger ketosis, and the reason for this is the operation of insulin. As soon as there is sufficient carbohydrate available (more than 60 g) the body reverts to the lazy option of using glucose and releasing insulin. There have been many studies looking at diets of 1200 calories with different quantities of carbohydrates, and as soon as you increase carbohydrate content above 60 g the body struggles to go into ketosis.

This is quite a well-known fact, but even today some researchers and experts fail or choose not to acknowledge it. In February 2009 the *New England Journal of Medicine* published a comparative study apparently showing that there was no difference between low-carb diets and traditional low-calorie, low-fat diets.[2] Unfortunately the researchers did not limit the starch and sugar content of the diet sufficiently, and therefore did not get the results that other comparative trials have shown. In fact, the fat content of the diet is irrelevant from a weight-loss perspective.

Another misunderstanding about ketosis is that some people say it is dangerous. The NHS website states:

Ketosis is a process in which your body converts fats into energy. During the conversion, ketones are produced as a by-product. Ketones can give your breath a sweet, fruity smell that may be mistaken for alcohol.

Your body normally uses glucose to meet its energy needs. Glucose comes from the carbohydrate in your diet. A healthy, balanced diet should provide you with all the glucose your body needs, so that ketosis does not take place. However, if your body does not have enough glucose, perhaps because your diet is very low in carbohydrates or you are starving yourself, it will begin ketosis to obtain energy from its stored fats instead. As a result of this, the ketone levels in your blood will rise. Prolonged severe ketosis can be dangerous as it can change the acidity of your blood, which may eventually lead to serious damage to your liver and kidneys.

Recently, diets that recommend you eat lots of protein and very little carbohydrate have become popular. These high-protein, low-carbohydrate diets, known as ketogenic diets, are intended to work by forcing your body to begin ketosis to burn fats and create quick weight loss. *Because long periods of ketosis can be dangerous to your kidneys and liver, ketogenic diets are never recommended by health professionals for more than short-term use, typically no longer than 14 days.* [My emphasis.] Many nutritionists warn their patients, especially women in the early stages of pregnancy, against following them at all.

It's a shame that the NHS writers have not bothered to read any of the peer-reviewed papers looking at the side effects of ketosis. You'll find a short list of the significant papers published that completely refute the fourteen-day warning in the notes to this chapter.[3] I have written to the NHS asking for the scientific basis of this warning but as yet they have not replied.

As these and other studies have shown, there is absolutely nothing unnatural about ketosis, nor is there anything dangerous. We are designed to go in and out of ketosis using real food or extreme exercise but we are not designed to live off shakes

Is it not strange that as we sit in the midst of a raging obesity crisis and have within our own bodies a natural solution, our experts really would rather people ate a diet that didn't work or took a drug or went under the knife? How mad is that unless you are a low-calorie food business or a drug company?

An in-depth article was printed in *The Business Magazine* in 2007 showing the financial benefits to drug companies of anti-obesity drugs. The obesity market is thought to be worth as much as $20 billion to the drug companies. Who wouldn't want to get in on the act? Alli, the over-the-counter version of Xenical, is said to be worth as much to GlaxoSmithKline as Nicorette, one of their major consumer products. Unfortunately many of the prescription drugs, like Reductil and others, have had a series of problems ranging from lawsuits to deaths. The market is huge and growing. In 2009, the NHS trust covering the city of Edinburgh spent £400,000 on diet drugs alone which was an increase of £395,000 from ten years ago.

So, for literally hundreds of thousands of years man happily went in and out of ketosis to deal with feast and famine. What is the problem? It would save the NHS thousands of pounds and would put control of the body back into the hands of the individual.

Unlike a low-calorie diet that almost requires a food technologist to tell you how many calories you are really eating, a low-carb diet requires no food technology intervention. Simply eat your natural diet without lots of fruit and, bingo, you are there. Once you are in ketosis there are several benefits that low-calorie diets cannot give you.

First, there is a real and tangible reduction in hunger. There has been much discussion over why satiety is so profound on a ketogenic diet. Some have argued that it is simply because of the high levels of protein, and others have suggested that once the body starts burning fat it no longer needs glucose and therefore no longer craves food. Others suggest that boredom is the key to satiety, but as yet there has never been evidence to support this argument. There is also an interesting argument that insulin is a key to hunger and when you reduce your insulin requirement, as you do when you are on a low-carb, high-protein diet, you also reduce hunger. Whatever the reason is, the outcome is the same. Hunger is simply not an issue when you are on a ketogenic diet.

Second, ketogenic diets can also help diabetics regulate their insulin requirements. In some cases type 2 diabetics can actually manage their diabetes without the need for drugs (though please take medical advice before stopping medication if this applies to you). This is probably the most shocking fact. With a diabetes epidemic in full swing we are busy prescribing drugs to solve a problem which diet alone could sort.

Third, ketogenic diets have been shown to improve cholesterol profiles of subjects. This was shown quite conclusively in the review by Hession.[4]

If there could be said to be one criticism of ketogenic diets, it's that for a short time (perhaps two to three days) you can feel a loss of concentration or tiredness while the body switches its energy source from starch and carbohydrates to body fat.

Surely now we must look again at this, a real obesity solution.

Summing up

Ketosis is a natural state for the human body

There are three ways to trigger ketosis and starvation (a very low-calorie diet is only one of the options). You can trigger ketosis by simply cutting out unnecessary starch and sugary foods, and still get all the nutrients you need for a healthy life.

Ketosis is safe when you follow a low-sugar/starch, high-protein real food option.

Ketosis does not require medical supervision when you follow the low-sugar/starch, high-protein real food option, and is a cheaper solution for obesity for the state than medication or surgery.

The modern hunter-gatherer

In the year 2010 when most of us in the West are not living like peasants, we need to move towards a diet which reflects our nutritional and lifestyle needs whether we are overweight or not. Put simply, the requirement for starch no longer exists in our modern lifestyle. In the modern world the issues are not starvation or energy-dense food, they are nutrition, health and obesity. The message of our government is stuck in the nineteenth century. Wake up – we are now in the third millennium!

Those of us who are overweight need a diet that will help us shed fat without losing muscle and which will, at the same time, ensure good health. Without doubt the real-food, ketogenic diet can do this sustainably.

Those of us who are lucky enough not to need a fat-loss solution need a diet that will energise us but be rich in nutrients to help us build healthy strong bodies without gaining fat. So what we want and need is a diet that reflects our individual needs.

Table 8.1 sets out a simple solution and shows how we should make food choices according to our health and lifestyle. The diet choices are based on the hunter-gatherer diets that we have evolved to eat, with some modern twists that have been brought into the human diet over the past 10,000 years and which, in moderation, are good for us – depending on our lifestyle. You'll find more information on dairy and pulses in the notes for this chapter.[1]

So the key message is to choose your diet to match your lifestyle and health profile. The simplistic message of one size fits all is simply garbage, even if it is an easy message to give to the public. Table 8.1 is the 'meatwell' guide on how to choose your diet!

	Protein (meat, fish, eggs)	Fresh green vegetables	Nuts and seeds	Fruit	Pulses	Dairy	Starch
Athlete	yes	yes	yes	yes	yes	yes	yes
Manual worker	yes	yes	yes	yes	yes	yes	yes
Naturally slim – no exercise required	yes	yes	yes	yes	yes	yes	yes
Slightly overweight	yes	yes	yes	Not during inch loss	Not during inch loss	yes	Not during inch loss. Always eat in moderation unless you take up lots of exercise – and I mean a lot.
Overweight /obese	yes	yes	yes	Limited amounts and low-GI choices after inch loss.	After inch loss	yes	After inch loss in limited quantities, but try to give it up as you don't need it.
Type 2 diabetics	yes	yes	yes	Yes – limited amounts after diabetes is under control	Limited amounts after diabetes is under control	yes	Give it up – you don't need it

Table 8.1 – Food choices

So whether you are thin or fat, athletic or not, the main part of your diet should be in the first four food columns. After that you need to make more difficult choices according to what you do and what you want to achieve.

You will note that there is no mention of sugar in Table 8.1. Frankly, sugar is not very useful at all. We get sugar from fruit and vegetables in abundance, and while a few may consider honey as a critical part of our diet it should be seen as an occasional luxury to be enjoyed only as a treat.

For type 2 diabetics, starch has really no benefit – but for the athlete a load of starch is perfectly fine. For computer geeks, there is little point filling up on starch since they are only using their fingers to tap a keyboard; it is far better to load up on protein, vegetables and fruit for the inactive, thinking lifestyle.

In response to the eatwell plate, here is the meatwell plate:

The Meatwell Plate

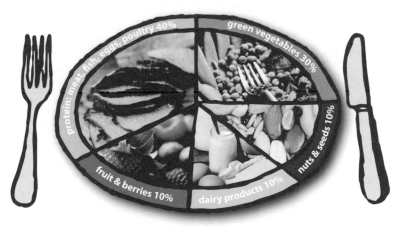

Figure 8.1 – The meatwell plate

FREEDOM FROM COUNTING ANYTHING

For the past thirty years we have been told to count calories. For others it is points, and for some it is fat grams. All this counting is not only stressful; it is misleading too. We know it is misleading from all the scientific studies reported in this book but, far worse than that, it is basically unsustainable without reliance on food manufacturers and that cannot be a good thing.

We need to stop the food scientists interfering with our relationship with food and making us reliant on them to manage our weight or health problems. We need to return to a simple understanding of whole foods. Wherever possible think like a hunter-gatherer. Was it there 10,000 years ago? If it wasn't, stop. Think 'Why would I want this? Is my body really designed to eat this? What will it do for me?'

Once you adopt this approach to food you no longer have to think about calories and other irrelevant information. A protein-rich diet will stop you eating too much, and a diet rich in green vegetables, nuts, seeds and berries will definitely give you enough vitamins and minerals to satisfy any nutritionist.

Liberate yourself from labelling and traffic lights and numbers.

Summing up

The meatwell guide allows you to make simple choices to fit your health and lifestyle.

The meatwell guide promotes diets which are rich in all the essentials, for a healthy body.

Liberate yourself from measuring food by numbers. Think about the food and its taste rather than its calorie or fat-gram volume. As shown, calorie counting has not helped us at all and, if anything, it has made us fat.

Think like a hunter-gatherer and you will never need to diet again.

Practical solutions

9

To lose excess fat efficiently and sustainably
you need to eat real food (not meal-
replacement shakes) and build up a way of
eating that can last a lifetime. The real-food,
ketogenic route provides just this. You begin your
journey eating just meat, fish, eggs and other protein
with some nuts, seeds, fruit and vegetables. You finish
with a broader range of foods. Here is the simple three-point plan:

STAGE ONE
Build your day around protein, adding the following:
◆ One handful of berries
◆ One handful of green vegetables (other than peas)
◆ Two handfuls of nuts (almonds, walnuts, brazil nuts) or seeds
◆ One glass of full-fat milk – with coffee and tea, or with your nuts and
  seeds as a home-made granola. People with lactose intolerance
  should use unsweetened soya milk instead.

This regime will put you into ketosis.

STAGE TWO
Continue this regime until you have nearly reached your goal size. Now
start introducing some more variety. In addition to the nuts, fruit and
vegetables above add the following:
◆ One extra handful of fruit (an apple or pear or tomato)
◆ One extra handful of vegetables
◆ One extra glass of milk, or perhaps a glass of red wine
◆ One square of dark chocolate (minimum 70% cocoa solids; read the
  label).

Once you are in ketosis your body will do most of the work but you do need to continue to eat as advised.

STAGE THREE

You are now at your target size and your goal is to add certain other foods to help you expand your menu to make it more enjoyable for the rest of your life. Each week you add one more of the following categories to your diet. Do not overdo it as this may cause your insulin levels to rise again and get you back to gaining fat.

◆ One handful of fruit
◆ One handful of green leafy vegetables
◆ One portion of pulses.

For recipes and more advice go to www.bigfatlies.co.uk.

THE TYPE 2 DIABETES SOLUTION

For type 2 diabetics, the simple solution for the silent killer is to stop eating foods that trigger a consistent need for insulin. Follow the stages below and watch not only your weight drop but also how your diabetes appears to fall away. In a recent study published in *Annals of Internal Medicine* (a publication by the American College of Physicians) the low carb diet led to more favourable changes in glycaemic control and coronary risk factors and delayed the need for drug therapy in overweight patients with newly diagnosed type 2 diabetes.[1]

STAGE ONE

Build your day around protein, adding the following:

◆ One handful of berries
◆ One handful of green vegetables (other than peas)
◆ Two handfuls of nuts (almonds, walnuts, brazil nuts) or seeds
◆ One glass of full-fat milk or unsweetened soya milk – with coffee and tea, or with your nuts and seeds as a home made granola.

This regime will put you into ketosis. This is not ketoacidosis; we mustn't confuse the two terms.

STAGE TWO

Continue this regime until you have nearly reached your goal size. Now start introducing some more variety. In addition to the nuts, fruit and vegetables above add the following:

◆ One extra handful of fruit (an apple or pear or tomato)
◆ One extra handful of vegetables
◆ One extra glass of milk, or perhaps a glass of red wine
◆ One square of dark chocolate (minimum 70% cocoa solids; read the label).

STAGE THREE

You are now at your target size and your goal is to add certain other foods to help you expand your menu to make it more enjoyable for the rest of your life. Each week you add one more of the following categories to your diet. Do not overdo it as this may cause your insulin levels to rise again and get you back to gaining fat.

◆ One portion of pulses
◆ One handful of fruit
◆ One handful of green leafy vegetables.

As before, visit www.bigfatlies.co.uk for recipes and more advice.

Summing up

Eat a pure hunter-gatherer diet for rapid weight loss.

As you lose the weight, evolve your diet towards one which includes further choices.

Accept that starch is unnecessary and will, in abundance, make you fat again.

Enjoy real food without worrying about volume again.

To you the jury

At the beginning of this book I explained how I went from law to nutrition because of two very simple questions: how do we become fat and how do we lose (or burn) fat? I also explained that while I am not a nutritionist, I am trained to ask questions and keep digging until I get a robust answer. Lawyers have always played a role in society of uncovering the truth through asking questions regardless of their own expertise. A lawyer's job is not to be an expert, but to expose lies.

The answers to both my questions are not simple because the human body is not simple. We are not combustion engines that simply require fuel and a little oil and a drive around the block. We are very complex.

Over the past thirty years the government has given us a one-dimensional message about losing weight, a message which has three parts:
◆ Eat less – eat fewer calories.
◆ Eat a balanced diet based on starch but low on saturated fat and sugar
◆ Do more exercise.

In other words, people are fat because they are greedy (either eating too much or too much of the wrong things) and lazy.

During this time more and more of us have become obese and the speed of obesity growth is accelerating. At the same time we know that we are trying to do what we are being told by the government because we are eating less, we are counting more calories, we are increasing our starch intake, we are reducing our fat and sugar intake and we are doing more exercise.

If this was a private company with poor financial results and the board of directors kept doing the same thing they would be sacked and sued. But things are less demanding for the government.

We know that the 'eat less, do more' message is being listened to but it is not working and it is not working because it is the wrong message. This incorrect message is making us fat.

◆ Counting calories does not work and there are studies to prove that
◆ Starch actually makes many of us fat. It operates like sugar in the body
◆ Exercise has very little effect on weight loss unless you do a huge amount or take up manual labour for six full days a week, every week.

The government could not have got it more wrong and is directly responsible for increasing the obesity problem in the UK. You are not fat because you are lazy and greedy, you are fat because you are eating a diet which is recommended by the government – and this diet and dietary advice is actually making you fat.

Fear of fat and love of starch has taken our government down a very dark blind alley and turning back and accepting this terrible mistake is no different to any other government cock-up. It is always hard to say 'we got it wrong' but the quicker the government accepts the mistake the better it will be for those who are obese or have diabetes. The quicker the government wises up to the metabolic effect of starch, the quicker we can turn this liner around and head away from icebergs towards sunnier climes.

Part of me would like to see an action for negligence raised against the government for this almighty mess, but mistakes are made. What is unforgivable is not to accept those mistakes when the evidence is there.

And as for the fear of saturated fats that has been promoted by the government, let's stop the stone-throwing and re-examine the apparently damning evidence again. We have sent people to their death on better evidence and still got it wrong. Whenever new evidence appears which questions the outcome of a murder trial we must not forget the prisoner in jail who may be innocent. If starch is to blame for the current health crisis, then perhaps saturated fats should be free and returned to its rightful place on our plate. What can be said with some certainty is that it is not a good idea to mix starch with saturated fats and then have a passive population.

Our evolutionary diet was a diet largely without starch but it did include saturated fats. So why make starch so important, especially when we know that modern hunter-gatherer tribes and ancient hunter-gatherer remains do not show signs of the modern diseases such as cancer or CVD? To ignore this evidence is indefensible in the current obesity crisis. The quicker we get back to our roots and embrace our natural diet, the quicker we have a chance of solving the obesity problem and ensuring that people eat a naturally nutrient-rich diet.

And as for exercise, I do hope someone, somewhere finally admits that asking people to solve their weight problem with exercise alone is really just a red herring!

Many of us are fat because of three big fat lies and now is the time to stop the bullshit and get on with really solving the problem – without blaming the British public for being lazy and greedy.

Appendix

CHAPTER 2

This was taken from a 2007 study – 'Obesity in Scotland, an Epidemiological Briefing' – looking in particular at obesity in Scotland but the findings remain true across the UK.

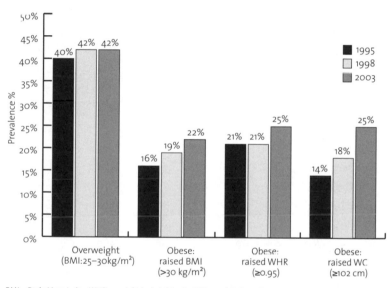

BMI = Body Mass Index; WHR = weight to height ratio; WC = waist circumference

Table 2.A – Prevalence of overweight and obesity in Scottish men, 16–64

	Proportion of men achieving physical activity guidelines	Proportion of women achieving physical activity guidelines
1997	32	21
1998	34	21
2003	36	24
2004	37	25

Table 2.B – Physical activity in the UK (source: The NHS Report, 2008)

CHAPTER 4

Essential Minerals Per 100 calorie portion	Sodium (Na), mg	Potassium (K), mg	Calcium (Ca), mg	Magnesium (Mg), mg	Phosphorus (P), mg
Biscuit, 1 (chocolate)	Trace	0	Trace	0	Trace
Bran Flakes, 40g (standard bowl) without fortification	320	240	16	48	180
Brazil nuts, 1.5	0.09	19.8	5.1	12.3	17.7
Egg, 1 (boiled)	70	65	28.5	6	100
Kidney beans, 100g (boiled)	2	420	37	45	130
New potatoes, 120g (boiled)	10.8	300	6	14.4	33.6
Spinach, 500g (boiled)	600	1150	800	170	140
Steak, 60g (grilled)	46.8	276	4.8	17.4	162
Strawberries, 36	19.8	528	52.8	33	79.2

Table 4.A – Essential minerals per 100 calorie portion

Iron (Fe), mg	Copper (Cu), mg	Zinc (Zn), mg	Chlorine (Cl), mg	Manganese (Mn), mg	Iodine (I), µg	Selenium (S), µg
0	0	0	0	0	0	0
This is added through fortification	0.14	1	524	0	0	(1.6)
0.075	0.0528	0.126	1.71	0.036	0.33	1.02
0.95	0.04	0.65	80	0	5.1	26.5
2.5	0.23	1	0	0.5	0	6
0.36	0.072	0.12	51.6	0	(3.6)	(1.2)
8	0.05	2.5	280	2.5	10	(5)
1.92	0.06	3.06	36.6	0.024	6.6	6
1.32	0.231	0.33	59.4	0.99	29.7	trace

Essential Vitamins Per 100 calorie portion	Vitamin A Retinol (µg)	Vitamin A Carotene (µg)	Vitamin D (µg)	Vitamin E (mg)
Biscuit, 1 (chocolate)	0	0	0	0
Bran Flakes, 40g (standard serving)	Added through fortification	Added through fortification	Added through fortification	Added through fortification
Brazil nuts, 1.5 (raw)	0	0	0	7.18
Egg, 1 (boiled)	95	Tr	0.9	0.555
Kidney beans, 100g (boiled)	0	4	0	0.20
New Potatoes, 120g (boiled)	0	Tr	0	(0.09)
Spinach, 500g (boiled)	0	33020	0	0
Steak, 60g (grilled)	Tr	5	0.3	0.05
Strawberries, 36 (raw)	0	26.4	0	0.66

Table 4.B – Essential vitamins (without industrialised fortification) per 100 calories

Thiamine B1, (mg)	Riboflavin B2, (mg)	Niacin B3, (mg)	Vitamin B6, (mg)	Vitamin B12, (μg)	Folate (μg)	Vitamin C (ascorbic acid, mg)
0	0	0	0	0	0	0
Added through fortification	Added through fortification	Added through fortification	Added through fortification	Added through fortification	Added through fortification	Added through fortification
0.67	0.03	0.3	0.31	0	0	0
0.035	0.175	0.05	0.06	0.55	19	0
0.17	0.05	0.6	0.12	0	42	1
0.108	0.072	2	0.432	0	21.6	18
0.3	0.25	4.5	0.45	0	405	40
0.8	0.21	5.1	0.5	2	4	0
0.099	0.099	1.98	0.198	0	66	254.1

Notes

CHAPTER 1

1. Brehm, B.J., Seeley, R.J., Daniels, S.R. et al., 'A Randomised Trial Comparing a Very Low Carbohydrate Diet and a Calorie-Restricted Low-Fat Diet.' *The Journal of Clinical Endocrinology and Metabolism*, 88(4), 2003, pp 1617–23

   Foster, G.D., Wyatt, H.R., Hill, J.O. et al., 'A Randomised Trial of a Low-Carbohydrate Diet for Obesity.' *The New England Journal of Medicine*, 348(21), 2003, pp 2082–90

   O'Brian, K.D., Brehm, B.J., Seeley, R.J., 'Greater Reduction in Inflammatory Markers with a Low-Carbohydrate Diet', Presented at American Heart Association's Scientific Sessions, 19 Nov 2002, Abstract ID 117597

   Samaha, F.F., Iqbal, N., 'A Low-Carbohydrate as Compared with a Low-Fat Diet in Severe Obesity.' *The New England Journal of Medicine*, 348(21), 2003, pp 2074–81

   Westman, E.C., Yancy, W.S., Edman, J.S. et al., 'Effect of Six-Month Adherence to a Very Low Carbohydrate Diet Program.' *The American Journal of Medicine*, July 2002, 113(1), pp 30–6

CHAPTER 2

1. The definition of obese is someone with a BMI of more than 30. The definition of overweight is someone with a BMI of more than 27. While it is true that these calculations have limited value in telling us how fat or unhealthy someone is, they do show us the scale of the problem and are still the main basis of statistics gathered in the UK.
2. The Information Centre Statistics on Obesity, Physical Activity and Diet in England, January 2008, otherwise known as the NHS Report 2008.
3. Haffner, S., 'Abdominal Obesity, Insulin Resistance and Cardiovascular Risk in Pre-Diabetes and Type 2 Diabetes, *European Heart Journal Supplement*, 2006

Yusuf, S. et al., 'Effect of Potentially Modifiable Risk Factors Associated with Myocardial Infarction in 52 Countries (the INTERHEART study), Case control study.' *Lancet*, 2004, 364 (9438) pp 937–52

4. Boyko, E. et al., 'Visceral Adiposity and the Risk of Type 2 Diabetes: A Prospective Study among Japanese Americans.' *Diabetes Care*, April 2000

5. The Early Bird Study is being undertaken by Professor Wilkin et al. of the Peninsula Medical School, Plymouth.

CHAPTER 3

1. http://www.eatwell.gov.uk/healthydiet

CHAPTER 4

1. Brehm, B.J et al., 'A Randomised Trial...' *The Journal of Clinical Endocrinology and Metabolism*, 2003

    Foster, G.D. et al., 'A Randomised Trial...' *The New England Journal of Medicine*, 2003

    O'Brian, K.D. et al., 'Greater Reduction ...', American Heart Association's Scientific Sessions, 2002

    Samaha, F.F., Iqbal, N., 'A Low-Carbohydrate as Compared ...' *The New England Journal of Medicine*, 2003

    Westman, E.C. et al., 'Effect of Six-Month Adherence...' *The American Journal of Medicine*, July 2002, 113(1), pp 30–6

2. Department of Health Report, 'Forecasting Obesity to 2010', July 2006 The Information Centre Statistics... January 2008.

3. Yusuf, S. et al., 'Effect of Potentially Modifiable Risk Factors... *Lancet*, 2004, 364 (9438) pp 937–52

4. Holt, S.H.A., Brand-Miller, J., Petocz, P. 'An Insulin Index of Foods: the Insulin Demand Generated by 1000-kJ Portions of Common Foods.' *American Journal of Clinical Nutrition*, 1997, 66, pp 1264–76.

5. Weigle, D.S. et al., 'A High-Protein Diet Induces Sustained Reductions in Appetite.' *American Journal of Clinical Nutrition*, 2005, pp 8241–8

Roll, B.J. et al., 'The Specificity of Satiety: The Influence of Foods of Different Macronutrient Content on the Development of Satiety.' *Physical Behaviour*, 1988

Astrup, A et al., 'Atkins and Other Low-Carbohydrate Diets: Hoax or an Effective Tool for Weight Loss?' *Lancet*, 2004, 364, pp 897–9

6. Trivedi, B., 'The Calorie Delusion.' *New Scientist*, 18 July 2009

7. Astrup, A. et al., 'Meta-Analysis of Resting Metabolic Rate in Formally Obese Subjects.' *American Journal of Clinical Nutrition*, 1999, 69, pp 1117–22

   Weinster, R.L. et al., 'Do Adaptive Changes in Metabolic Rate Favour Weight Regain in Weight-Reduced Individuals?' *American Journal of Clinical Nutrition*, 2000, 72 pp 1088–94

   Wadden, T.A. et al., 'Relationship of Dietary History to Resting Metabolic Rate, Body Composition, Eating Behaviour And Subsequent Weight Loss.' *American Journal of Clinical Nutrition*, 1992

8. Kondepudi, D., Prigogine, I., *Modern Thermodynamics: From heat engines to dissipative structures*, Wiley and Sons, 1998

9. Buchholz, A.C., Schoeller, D.A., 'Is a Calorie a Calorie?' *American Journal of Clinical Nutrition*, 2004, 79 (suppl), pp 899s-906s

10. Dyson, P.A. et al., 'A Low-Carbohydrate Diet is More Effective in Reducing Body Weight than Healthy Eating in both Diabetic and Non-Diabetic Subjects.' *Diabetic Medicine*, 2007, D01 10.1111

    Dyson, P.A., 'A Review of Low- and Reduced-Carbohydrate Diets and Weight Loss in Type 2 Diabetes.' *Journal of Human Nutrition and Dietetics*, 2008

    Hession, M. et al., 'Systematic Review of Randomized Controlled Trials of Low-Carbohydrate Versus Low-Fat/Low-Calorie Diets in the Management of Obesity and its Comorbidities.' *Obesity*, 2008

11. Harper A.E. 'Defining the essentiality of nutrients' in *Modern Nutrition in Health and Disease*, 9th edition. M. E. Shils, J. A. Olsen, M. Shike and A. C. Ross (editors), Baltimore: Williams & Wilkins, 1999

12. Holt, S.H., Miller, J.C., and Petocz, P., 'An insulin index of foods: the insulin demand generated by 1000-kJ portions of common foods', *American Journal of Clinical Nutrition*, 1997, 66, pp 1264–76

13. Holt, S.H., Miller, J.C., and Petocz, P., 'An insulin index of foods: the insulin demand generated by 1000-kJ portions of common foods', *American Journal of Clinical Nutrition*, 1997, 66, pp 1264–76

14. Larsson, S.C. et al., 'Glycemic Load, Glycemic Index and Breast Cancer Risk in a Prospective Cohort of Swedish Women.' *International Journal of Cancer*, 2009; 125 (1): pp 153–7

15. Gunter, M.J. et al., Insulin, Insulin-Like Growth Factor-1 and the Risk of Breast Cancer in Post-Menopausal Women.' *Journal of the National Cancer Initiative*, 2008

16. Lajour, M. et al., 'Carbohydrate Intake, Glycaemic Index, Glycaemic Load and the Risk of Postmenopausal Breast Cancer in a Prospective Study of French Women.' *American Journal of Clinical Nutrition*, 2008: 87, pp 1384–91

17. Freeland, S. et al., 'Restriction of Carbohydrates and Prostate Tumour Growth.' *Cancer Prevention Research*, 26 May 2009

18. Leibowitz, S.F. at al., 'Acute High-Fat Diet Paradigms Link Galanin to Triglycerides and their Transport and Metabolism in Muscle.' *Brain Research*, 2004, 1008, 168–78
Romon, M. et al., 'Leptin Response to Carbohydrate or Fat Meals and Association with Subsequent Satiety and Energy Intake.' *American Physiological Society*, 1999

19. Cordain, L. et al., 'The Paradoxical Nature of Hunter-Gatherer Diets: Meat-based yet Non-Atherogenic.' *European Journal of Clinical Nutrition*, 2002, 56 (suppl1) pp s42-s52

20. Brehm, B.J et al., 'A Randomised Trial...' *The Journal of Clinical Endocrinology and Metabolism*, 2003
Foster, G.D. et al., 'A Randomised Trial...' *The New England Journal of Medicine*, 2003
Mozaffarian, D. et al., 'Dietary Fats, Carbohydrate and Progression of Coronary Atherosclerosis in Postmenopausal Women.' *American Journal of Clinical Nutrition*, 2004, 80(5), pp 1175–84
O'Brian, K.D. et al., 'Greater Reduction ...', American Heart Association's Scientific Sessions, 2002
Samaha, F.F., Iqbal, N., 'A Low-Carbohydrate as Compared ...' *The New England Journal of Medicine*, 2003
Westman, E.C. et al., 'Effect of Six-Month Adherence...' *The American Journal of Medicine*, July 2002, 113(1), pp 30–6

21. Information from the European Heart Network and the British Heart Foundation.

22. Ascherio, A. et al., 'Dietary Fat and Risk of Coronary Heart Disease in Men: Cohort Follow-Up Study in the United States.' *British Medical Journal*, 1996, 313, pp 84–90

Dolecek, T.A., Epidemiological Evidence of Relationships Between Dietary Polyunsaturated Fatty Acids and Mortality in The Multiple Risk Factor Intervention Trial.' *Proceedings of the Society for Experimental Biology and Medicine*, 1992, 200(2), pp 177–82

Farchi, G. et al., 'Diet And 20-Year Mortality in Two Rural Population Groups of Middle-Aged Men in Italy.' *American Journal of Clinical Nutrition*, 1989, 50(5), pp 1095–1103

Fehily, A.M. et al., 'Diet and Incident Ischemic Heart Disease: the Caerphilly Study.' *British Journal of Nutrition*, 1993, 69, pp 303–14

Garcia-Palmieri, M.R. et al., 'Relationship of Dietary Intake to Subsequent Coronary Heart Disease Incidence: The Puerto Rico Heart Health Program.' *American Journal of Clinical Nutrition*, 1980, 33(8), pp 1818–27

Goldbourt, U. et al., 'Factors Predictive of Long-Term Coronary Heart Disease Mortality Among 10,059 Male Israeli Civil Servants and Municipal Employees: A 23-Year Mortality Follow-Up in the Israeli Ischemic Heart Disease Study.' *Cardiology*, 1993, 82, pp 100–21

Gordon, T., *The Framingham Diet Study: Diet and the Regulation of Serum Cholesterol in the Framingham Study; An Epidemiological Investigation of Cardiovascular Disease*, Section 24, US Government Printing Office, Washington DC, 1970

Gordon, T, et al., 'Diet and its Relation to Coronary Heart Disease in Three Populations.' *Circulation*, 1981, 63, pp 500-15

Hu, F.B. et al., 'Dietary Fat Intake and the Risk of Coronary Heart Disease in Women.' *New England Journal of Medicine*, 1997, 337 (21), pp 1491–9

Khaw, K. T. et al., 'Dietary Fiber and Reduced Ischemic Heart Disease Mortality Rates in Men and Women: A 12-Year Prospective Study.' *American Journal of Epidemiology*, 1987, 126 (6), pp 1093–1102

Kromhout, D. et al., 'Diet, Prevalence and Ten-Year Mortality from Coronary Heart Disease in 871 Middle-Aged Men: The Stephen Study.' *American Journal of Epidemiology*, 1984, 119, pp 733–41

Laaksonen, D.E. et al., 'Prediction of Cardiovascular Mortality in Middle-Aged Men by Dietary and Serum Linoleic And Polyunsaturated Fatty Acids.' *Archives of Internal Medicine*, 2005, 165, pp 193–9

Lapidus, L. et al., 'Dietary Habits in Relation to Incidence of Cardiovascular Disease and Death in Women: A 12-Year Follow-Up of Participants in the Population Study of Women in Gothenburg, Sweden.' *American Journal of Clinical Nutrition*, 1986, 44(4), pp 444–8

Leosdottir, M. et al., 'Dietary Fat Intake and Early Mortality Patterns – Data from the Malmo Diet and Cancer Study.' *Journal of Internal Medicine*, 2005, 258, pp 153–65

Meddalie, J.H. et al., 'Five-Year Myocardial Infarction Incidence 11 – Association of Single Variables to Age and Birthplace.' *Journal of Chronic Diseases*, 1973, 26(6), pp 325–49

Morris, I.N. et al., 'Diet and Heart: A Postscript.' *British Medical Journal*, 1977, 2 pp 1307–14

Paul, O. et al., 'A Longitudinal Study of Coronary Heart Disease.' *Circulation Journal*, 1963, 963:28, pp 20–31

Pietinen, P. et al., 'Intake of Fatty Acids and Risk of Coronary Heart Disease in a Cohort of Finnish Men: The Alpha–Tocopherol, Beta–Carotene Cancer Prevention Study.' *American Journal of Epidemiology*, 1997, 145, pp 876–87

Posner, B. M. et al., 'Dietary Lipid Predictors of Coronary Heart Disease in Men: The Framingham Study' *Archives of Internal Medicine*, 1991, 151, pp 1181–7

Shekelle, R.B. et al., 'Diet, Serum Cholesterol and Death From Coronary Heart Disease: The Western Electric Study.' *New England Journal of Medicine*, 1981, 304, pp 65–70

Tanasescu, M. et al., 'Dietary Fat and Cholesterol and the Risk of Cardiovascular Disease Among Women with Type 2 Diabetes.' *American Journal of Clinical Nutrition*, 2004, 79, pp 999–1005

Yano, K. et al., 'Dietary Intake and the Risk of Coronary Heart Disease in Japanese Men Living in Hawaii.' *American Journal of Clinical Nutrition*, 1978, 31, pp 1270–9

Esrey, K.L. et al., 'Relationship Between Dietary Intake and Coronary Heart Disease Mortality: Lipid Research Clinics Prevalence Follow-Up Study, *Journal of Clinical Epidemiology*, 1996, 49(2), pp 211–16

Kushi, L. H. et al., Diet and 20-Year Mortality from Coronary Heart Disease: The Ireland–Boston Diet–Heart Study.' *New England Journal of Medicine*, 1985, 312, pp 811–18

McGee, D.L. et al., 'Ten-Year Incidence of Coronary Heart Disease in the Honolulu Heart Program: Relationship to Nutrient Intake.' *American Journal of Epidemiology*, 1984, 119, pp 667–76

Tucker, K.L. et al., 'The Combination of High Fruit and Vegetable and Low-Saturated Fat Intakes is More Protective against Mortality in Ageing Men than is Either Alone: the Baltimore Longitudinal Study of Aging.' *Journal of Nutrition*, 2005, 135, pp 556–61

23. American Heart Association, 'National Diet Heart Study Final Report', *Circulation*, 1968, 37:3 (supplement) pp 1–419

'Controlled Trial of Soya Bean Oil in Myocardial Infarction.' *Lancet*, 1968, 2(7570), pp 693–9

Bierenbaum, M.L. et al., 'Modified Fat Dietary Management of the Young Male with Coronary Disease: A Five-Year Report.' *Journal of the American Medical Association*, 1967, 202(13), pp 1119–23

Burr, M.L. et al., 'Effects Of Changes in Fat, Fish and Fibre Intakes on Death and Myocardial Reinfarction: Diet And Reinfarction Trial (DART).' *Lancet*, 1989, 2(8666), pp 757–61

Christakis, G. et al., 'Effect of the Anti-Coronary Club on Coronary Heart Disease Risk Factor Status.' *Journal of the American Medical Association*, 1966, 198(6), pp 597–604

Hjermann, I. et al., 'Effect of Diet and Smoking in the Incidence of Coronary Heart Disease.' *Lancet*, 1981, II, pp 1303–10

Howard, B.V. et al., 'Low-Fat Dietary Pattern and Risk of Cardiovascular Disease: The Women's Health Initiative Randomized Controlled Dietary Modification Trial.' *Journal of the American Medical Association*, 2006, 295, pp 655–66

Key, T.J. et al., 'Dietary Habits and Mortality in 11,000 Vegetarians and Health-Conscious People: Results of a 17-Year Follow-Up.' *British Medical Journal*, 1996, 313, pp 775–9

Key, T.J, et al., 'Mortality in British Vegetarians: Review and Preliminary Results from the EPIC Study.' *American Journal of Clinical Nutrition*, 2003, 78 (suppl), pp 533s–538s

Leren, P., 'The Oslo Diet Heart Study: Eleven-Year Report.' *Circulation*, 1970, 42:935

De Lorgeril, M. et al., 'Mediterranean Alpha-Linolenic-Acid-Rich Diet in Secondary Prevention of Coronary Heart Disease, *Lancet*, 1994, 343(8911), pp 1454–9

Miettinen, M. et al., 'Effect of Cholesterol-lowering Diet on Mortality from Coronary Heart Disease and Other Causes: A Twelve-Year Clinical Trial in Men and Women.' *Lancet*, 1972, 2 (7782), pp 835–8

Neaton, J.D. et al., 'Serum Cholesterol Level and Mortality Findings for Men Screened in the Multiple Risk Fact Intervention Trial.' *Archives of Internal Medicine* 1992, 152, pp 1490–1500

Rose, G.A. et al., 'Corn Oil in the Treatment of Ischaemic Heart Disease.' *British Medical Journal*, 1965, pp 1531–3

Strandberg, T.E. et al., 'Long-Term Mortality After Five Years: Multifactorial Primary Prevention of Cardiovascular Diseases in Middle-Aged Men.' *Journal of the American Medical Association*, 1991, 266: 1229

Thorogood, M. et al., 'Risk of Death from Cancer and Ischemic Heart Disease in Meat and Non-Meat Eaters.' *British Medical Journal*, 1994, 308, pp 1667–70

Turpenien, O. et al., 'Dietary Prevention of Coronary Heart Disease: The Finnish Mental Hospital Study.' *International Journal of Epidemiology*, 1979, 8, pp 9-118

Watts, G.F. et al., 'Effects on Coronary Artery Disease of Lipid Lowering Diet or Diet Plus Cholelstyramine in the St Thomas's Atherosclerosis Regression Study (STARS).' *Lancet*, 1992, 339 (8793), pp 563–9

Woodhill, J.M. et al., Low-fat, Low-Cholesterol Diet in Secondary Prevention of Coronary Heart Disease.' *Advances in Experimental Medicine and Biology*, 1978, 109, pp 317–30

World Health Organization European Collaborative Group, 'European Collaborative Trial of Multifactorial Prevention of Coronary Heart Disease.' *Lancet*, 1986, 1, pp 869–72

24. Dayton, S. et al., 'A Controlled Clinical Trial of a Diet High in Unsaturated Fat in Preventing Complications of Atherosclerosis.' *Circulation*, 1969, 40 (Suppl 11), pp 1–63

Frantz, I.D. Jr. et al., 'Test of Effect of Lipid Lowering by Diet on Cardiovascular Risk: The Minnesota Coronary Survey.' *Arteriosclerosis*, 1989, 9, pp 129–35

25. Howard, B.V. et al., 'Low-Fat Dietary Pattern...' *Journal of the American Medical Association*, 2006, 295, pp 655–66

26. Mozaffarian, D. et al., 'Dietary Fats, Carbohydrate...' *American Journal of Clinical Nutrition*, 2004

27. Edefonti, V. et al., 'Nutrient Dietary Patterns and the Risk of Breast and Ovarian Cancers.' *International Journal of Cancer*, 2008, 122(3), pp 609–613

28. Lawson, L.D. et al., 'Beta-Oxidation of The Coenzyme A Esters of Elaidic, Oleic and Stearic Acids and their Full-Cycle Intermediates by Rat Heart Mitochondria.' *International Journal of Biochemistry, Biophysics and Molecular Biology*, 1979, 573, pp 245–54

29. Hooper, L. et al., 'Dietary Intake and Prevention of Cardiovascular Disease Systematic Review.' *British Medical Journal*, 2001, 322 (7289), pp 757–63

30 Yusuf, S. et al., 'Effect of Potentially Modifiable Risk Factors...' *Lancet*, 2004

31. Dietary and Nutritional Survey of British Adults, 1986–1987, Office of Population Censuses and Surveys, Social Survey Division, MAFF. The purpose of this survey was to produce data on the food and nutrient intake, nutritional status, anthropometric and blood-pressure measurements of the British population aged between 16 and 64 in 1986–7.

32. Sigman, G.M., 'Can You Have Your Low-Fat Cake and Eat it Too?' *Journal of the American Dietetic Association*, 1997, Supplement S76

33. Talbot, G., 'Independent Advice on Possible Reductions for Saturated Fat in Products that Contribute to Consumer Intakes.' Summary report prepared for the FSA, November 2006.

34. Ongoing Early Bird Study.

35. Turpenien, O. et al., 'Dietary Prevention...' *International Journal of Epidemiology*, 1979

36. Swinburn, B., 'Increased Energy Intake Alone Virtually Explains All the Increase in Body Weight in the United States from 1970s to the 2000s.' *European Congress on Obesity 2009 Abstract*, Ti Rs3.3

37. Duclos, M. et al., 'Acute and Chronic Effects of Exercise on Tissue Sensitivity to Glucocorticoids.' *Journal of Applied Physiology*, 2003, 94, pp 867-75

38. Fraser, R. et al., 'Cortisol Effects on Body Mass, Blood Pressure and Cholesterol in the General Population.' *Hypertension*, 1999, p 1365

CHAPTER 5

1. Brehm, B.J et al., 'A Randomised Trial...' *The Journal of Clinical Endocrinology and Metabolism*, 2003

    Claessens, M. et al., 'The Effect of a Low-Fat, High-Protein or High-Carbohydrate ad libitum Diet on Weight-Loss Maintenance and Metabolic Risk Factors.' *International Journal of Obesity*, 2009, pp 1–9

    Dyson, P.A. et al., 'A Low-Carbohydrate Diet is More Effective in Reducing Body Weight than Healthy Eating in both Diabetic and Non-Diabetic Subjects.' *Diabetic Medicine*, 2007, D01 10.1111

    Foster, G.D. et al., 'A Randomised Trial...' *The New England Journal of Medicine*, 2003

    Hession, M. et al., 'Systematic review...' *Obesity*, 2008

    Kushner, R.F. et al., 'Low-carbohydrate, high-protein diets revisited.' *Gastroenterology*, 2008, 24, pp 198–203

    O'Brian, K.D. et al., 'Greater Reduction ...', American Heart Association's Scientific Sessions, 2002

    Samaha, F.F., Iqbal, N., 'A Low-Carbohydrate as Compared ...' *The New England Journal of Medicine*, 2003

    Shai, I. et al., 'Weight Loss with Low-Carbohydrate, Mediterranean, Low-Fat Diets.' *New England Journal of Medicine*, 2008, Vol 359, No 3

    Westman, E.C. et al, 'Effect of Six-Month Adherence...' *The American Journal of Medicine*, July 2002, 113(1), pp 30–6

CHAPTER 6

1. Cordain, L. et al., 'Fatty-Acid Composition and Energy Density of Foods Available to African Hominids: Evolutionary Implications for Human Brain Development.' *World Review of Nutrition*, 2001, 90, pp 144–61

    Stefansson, V., *The Fat of the Land*, New York, MacMillan, 1960, pp 15–39

2. Crawford, M.A. et al., 'A New Theory of Evolution: Quantum Theory.' *American Oil Chemists' Society*, 1992, pp 87–95

    Eaton, S.B., 'Humans, lipids and evolution.' *Lipids*, 1992, 27, pp 814–20

3. Cordain, L. et al., 'Plant–Animal Subsistence Ratios and Macronutrient Energy Estimations in Worldwide Hunter-Gatherer Diets.' *American Journal of Clinical Nutrition*, 2000, 71(3), pp 682–92
4. Dr Jay Stock, Department of Archaeology and Anthropology, University of Cambridge.
5. Diamond, J., 'The Worst Mistake in The History of the Human Race.' *Discover*, 1987, pp 64–6
6. Diamond, J: as above
7. Eaton, S.B., 'Fibre Intake in Prehistoric Times', in Leeds, A.R. (ed), *Dietary Fibre Perspectives 2, Reviews and Bibliography*, 1990 pp 27–40
8. Nolan, P., *Work in the Twenty-first Century; Demystifying the Weightless Economy*, Economic and Social Research Council, 2008
9. Carnoy, M., Castells, M., Cohen, S.S. and Cardoso, F.H., *The New Global Economy in the Information Age: Reflections on Our Changing World*, University Park, PA: Pennsylvania State University Press, 1993
10. Nolan, P., *Work in the Twenty-first Century...* Economic and Social Research Council, 2008
11. O'Keefe, J.H., Cordain, L., 'Cardiovascular Disease Resulting From a Diet and Lifestyle at Odds With Our Palaeolithic Genome: How to Become a 21st-Century Hunter-Gatherer.' *Mayo Clinic Proceedings*, 2004, 79 pp 101–8.
12. Cordain, L., Eaton, S.B., Miller, J.B., Mann, N., Hill, K. 'The Paradoxical Nature of Hunter-Gatherer Diets: Meat-based, yet non-atherogenic.' *European Journal of Clinical Nutrition*, 2002, 56 (suppl 1), pp s42–s52.
13. Eaton, S.B., Eaton, S.B, (III). Konner, M.J., 'Palaeolithic Nutrition Revisited: A Twelve-Year Retrospective on its Nature and Implications.' *European Journal of Clinical Nutrition*, 1997, 51, pp 207–16.
14. O'Keefe, J.H., Cordain, L., 'Cardiovascular Disease...' *Mayo Clinic Proceedings*, 2004
15. Cordain, L. et al., 'The Paradoxical Nature...' *European Journal of Clinical Nutrition*, 2002
16. Cordain, L. et al., 'The Paradoxical Nature...' *European Journal of Clinical Nutrition*, 2002
17. Eaton, S.B. et al., 'Palaeolithic Nutrition Revisited...' *European Journal of Clinical Nutrition*, 1997

18. Bowen, J., Noakes, M., Clifton, P.M. 'A High-Dairy, High-Calcium Diet Minimizes Bone Turnover in Overweight Adults during Weight Loss.' *Journal of Nutrition*, 2004, 134, pp 568–73.
19. Cordain, L. et al., 'The Paradoxical Nature...' *European Journal of Clinical Nutrition*, 2002
20. Bowen, J. et al., 'A High-Dairy, High-Calcium Diet...' *Journal of Nutrition*, 2004
21. Cordain, L., Eaton, B., Sebastian, A., Mann, N., Lindeberg, S., Watkins, B.A., O'Keefe, J.H., Brand-Miller, J., 'Origins and Evolution of the Western Diet: Health Implications for the 21st Century.' *Journal of Clinical Nutrition*, 2005, 81, pp 341–54.
22. Cordain, L. et al., 'Origins and Evolution...' *Journal of Clinical Nutrition*, 2005
23. Holt, S.H.A., Brand-Miller, J., Petocz, P., 'An Insulin Index of Foods...' *American Journal of Clinical Nutrition*, 1997.
24. Cordain, L. et al., 'Plant–Animal Subsistence Ratios ...' *American Journal of Clinical Nutrition,* 2000
    Milton, K., 'Hunter-Gatherer Diets – A Different Perspective.' *American Journal of Clinical Nutrition*, 2000, 71, pp 665–7
25. In the *European Journal of Clinical Nutrition*, 2009
26. Hession, M. et al., 'Systematic review...' *Obesity*, 2008
27. Bravata, Dena M., Sanders, L., Huang J. et al., 'Efficacy and Safety of Low-Carbohydrate Diets: A Systematic Review.' *Journal of the American Medical Association*, 9 April 2003, 9: 14, pp 1837–50
28. Brinkworth, G.D., Noakes, M., Keogh, J.B. et al., 'Long-Term Effects of a High-Protein, Low-Carbohydrate Diet on Weight Control and Cardiovascular Risk Markers in Obese Hyperinsulinemic Subjects.' *International Journal of Obesity*, 2004, 28: 5, pp 661–70.
29. Barnett, A.H., Kumar, S., eds, *Obesity and Diabetes*, Wiley, second edition 2009. The chapters have different authors; Professor Broom is particularly referring to the one he co-authored.
30. Kushner, R.F. et al., 'Low-carbohydrate...' *Gastroenterology*, 2008
31. Claessens, M. et al., 'The Effect of a Low-Fat, High-Protein or High-Carbohydrate ad libitum ...' *International Journal of Obesity*, 2009
32. Shai, I. et al., 'Weight Loss with Low-Carbohydrate...' *New England Journal of Medicine*, 2008, Vol 359, No 3

33. Dyson, P.A. et al., 'A Low-Carbohydrate Diet ...' *Diabetic Medicine*, 2007
34. Davis, N.J. et al., 'Comparative Study of the Effects of a One-Year Dietary Intervention of a Low-Carbohydrate Diet versus a Low-Fat Diet on Weight and Glycemic Control in Type 2 Diabetes.' *Diabetes Care*, 2009, 32
35. Hession, M. et al., 'Systematic review...' *Obesity*, 2008
36. Davis, N.J. et al., 'Comparative Study ...' *Diabetes Care*, 2009
37. Hession, M. et al., 'Systematic review...' *Obesity*, 2008
38. Frisch, S., Zittermann, A., Berthold, H.K., et al., 'A randomized controlled trial on the efficacy of carbohydrate-reduced or fat-reduced diets in patients attending a telemedically guided weight loss program.' *Cardiovascular Diabetology*, 2009, 8:36.
39. Sacks, F.M. et al., 'Comparison of Weight-Loss Diets with Different Compositions of Fat, Protein and Carbohydrates.' *New England Journal of Medicine*, 26 Feb 2009, vol. 360, no. 9

CHAPTER 7

1. Ketoacidosis is when someone with type 1 diabetes does not have enough insulin in their body for it to use the glucose in the blood to create energy. That then results in high blood-glucose levels, and this leads to dehydration as the body attempts to remove excess glucose by passing more urine. This, in turn, affects the level of electrolytes in the body. If left untreated, the body will release so many ketones into the blood that it will quickly become dangerously acidic. Together with unbalanced electrolyte levels and dehydration, untreated diabetic ketoacidosis can lead to coma and death.
2. Sacks, F.M. et al., 'Comparison of Weight Loss Diets...' *New England Journal of Medicine*, 2009, 360:9
3. Dashti, H.M. et al., 'Beneficial Effects of Ketogenic Diet in Obese Diabetic Subjects.' *Molecular and Cellular Biochemistry*, 2007, 10.1007/s11010-007-9448-z
   Shai, I. et al., 'Weight Loss with Low-Carbohydrate...' *New England Journal of Medicine*, 2008
   Hession, M. et al., 'Systematic review...' *Obesity*, 2008

Dyson, P.A., 'A Review of Low- and Reduced-Carbohydrate Diets and Weight Loss in Type 2 Diabetes.' *Journal of Human Nutrition and Dietetics*, 2008

Dyson, P.A. et al., 'A Low-Carbohydrate Diet...' *Diabetic Medicine*, 2007

4. Hession, M. et al., 'Systematic review...' *Obesity*, 2008

CHAPTER 8

1. Dairy is a key part of many people's diet today, but many dairy products such as cheese, butter and cream are fairly recent additions to the human diet. We may have had some cow or goat milk (full fat) but little else. Dairy is often high in fat and can be relatively high in protein. The history of dairy products and health is a little mixed. I certainly grew up believing that dairy was food for bones, but in fact the evidence for that is poor. The *Journal of Paediatrics* published a review study looking at the benefits of dairy and only ten out of thirty-seven studies showed a relationship between dairy intake and calcium and, of the ten that did show a link, the benefit was small (Lanou A. J. et al., 'Calcium, dairy products and bone helath in children and young adults: a re-evaluation of the evidence.' *Pediatrics*, 2005, 115:3, pp 736–43). *The British Medical Journal* also published a study reviewing evidence from nineteen studies looking at calcium supplements and yet again there seemed to be little evidence of improved bone density in the hip or spine and only marginal improvement in the arm (Winzenberg, T., et al., 'Effects of calcium supplementation on bone density in healthy children: meta-analysis of randomised controlled trials.' *British Medical Journal*, 2006, 333, pp 775–8).

    But what about the old? Again the evidence that dairy is great for bones is poor. The *American Journal of Clinical Nutrition* published a study analysing 72,000 women for eighteen years, trying to show a link between calcium intake and hip fractures (Feskanich, D., Willett, W.C. and Colditz, G.A. 'Calcium, vitamin D, milk consumption, and hip fractures: a prospective study among postmenopausal women.' *American Journal of Clinical Nutrition*, 2003, 77: 2 pp 504–11). Another review of literature found that only two of fourteen studies showed any relationship between milk consumption and bone health in women after the age of fifty (Weinsier, R.L. and Krumdieck, C.L. 'Dairy foods and bone health: examination of the evidence.' *American Journal of Clinical Nutrition*, 2000, 72, pp 681–9).

One of the challenges with dairy is that it has been linked to food intolerances and therefore eating dairy is really not an option for many people. But if you do decide to choose dairy products, then choose only those in their whole form. Avoid the low-fat options; they have been heavily processed.

Pulses are often seen as a superfood due to their fantastic balance between protein and carbohydrate. In many ways we know very little about these foods and they have only been part of our diet for 10,000 years which, in the world of diet, is really just a matter of minutes. In any event, many of us enjoy these foods and they are part of most people's diet. They are fine when you are not in weight-loss mode, and when you restrict the volume you eat depending on the amount of activity you do and your own insulin response to this carbohydrate food.

CHAPTER 9

1. Kelly et al., 'Systematic review: glucose control and cardiovascular disease in Type 2 diabetes', *Annals of Internal Medicine*. 2009. Volume 151, Issue 6.

Index